Suzy Prudden's Pregnancy & Back-to-shape Exercise Program

Suzy Prudden's Pregnancy & Back-to-shape Exercise Program

By Suzy Prudden and Jeffrey Sussman

Introductory comments by Dr. Alan Davidson and Dr. Howard R. Rappaport
Photographs by Maje Waldo

Workman Publishing, New York

Books by Suzy Prudden & Jeffrey Sussman

Creative Fitness For Baby & Child
Suzy Prudden's Family Fitness Book
Fit For Life
See How They Run
Suzy's Prudden's Spot Reducing Program

Library of Congress Cataloging in Publication Data

Prudden, Suzy.
   Suzy Prudden's Pregnancy and back-to-shape exercise program.
1. Pregnancy.   2. Exercise for women.
3. Prenatal care.   4. Postnatal care.
5. Infants—Care and hygiene.   6. Exercise for children.   I. Sussman, Jeffrey, joint author.
II. Title.   III. Title: Pregnancy and back-to-shape exercise program.
RG558.P78   618.2'4   80-51614
ISBN 0-89480-130-9
ISBN 0-89480-129-5 (pbk.)

Cover and book design: Charles Kreloff
Suzy Prudden's leotards of nylon with "Lycra" spandex by Capezio Ballet Makers

Manufactured in the United States of America
First printing November 1980

20 19 18 17 16 15 14 13 12 11 10 9

Workman Publishing Company, Inc.
708 Broadway
New York, New York 10003

Acknowledgements

In our previous book, *Suzy Prudden's Spot Reducing Program*, we expressed our gratitude to members of the staff of a unique publishing company, Workman. However, there are many others at Workman whose talents did not manifest themselves until after our book had been published. Therefore, we would like to take this opportunity to thank Christopher Power for his singular kindness and generosity, Bert Snyder for making sure that our book was in every city in every bookstore across the country, and Sallie Jackson for being such a friendly voice.

We would especially like to thank Jeremy Basescu, Trevor A. Fradkin, Jennifer Vogel, Andrea Victor and their mothers for their cooperation in photographing the Infant Starter exercises. A very special thanks goes to Carolyn Silberstein, the model for the Pregnancy section who gave birth to Matthew as this book went to press.

Dedication

To Donald and Flora Beckley, generous grandparents, and to our son, Robby, who inspired this book and so much more.

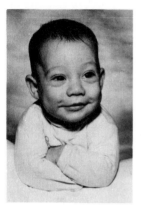

Robby Sussman, age 3 months

Introductory Comments

Suzy Prudden has been a pioneer in teaching exercise courses for pregnant women, and she has done a superb job in applying her years of practical experience to writing this book. It concisely outlines in words and pictures the essential exercises used to prepare your body for labor and delivery, and to allow you to rapidly return to tiptop physical condition.

Any program of exercise should be approved by the patient's doctor, since vaginal staining, heart or lung problems, or back conditions may be definite contra-indications for certain exercises. If there is any pain or discomfort, exercises should be immediately discontinued. If the pain persists, the patient should consult her physician. Good nutrition and the avoidance of excessive weight gain are an important part of any exercise program. Stretch marks may occur in any pregnancy, but may be partially avoided by Suzy Prudden's exercises.

I strongly recommend this book to anyone who takes pride in her body and desires to prepare it for labor and delivery, and for the post-partum period.

Alan Davidson, M.D.
Assistant Professor in Obstetrics and Gynecology, Mount Sinai School of Medicine
Associate Attending in Obstetrics and Gynecology, Mount Sinai Hospital, New York City

Introductory Comments

The name Suzy Prudden is well known to all who have an interest in "staying in shape." And now, Suzy Prudden has written an exercise book for infants. Will it do anything?

Pediatricians have always believed in prevention. It is an article of faith for us —vaccinations have erradicated smallpox from the world; diptheria and polio are also yielding to immunization. It now seems possible that even heart disease and cancer may be treated by early attention to diet and lifestyle.

A close look at the pictures in the Infant Starter section will reveal the value of Suzy's program. There is an intimacy and warmth, a touching and handling that you and your baby share that tells you your baby is not fragile, and is capable of responding to life. That sharing and awareness will make you a more confident parent, and that has to be beneficial to you and your baby.

Howard R. Rappaport, M.D.
Assistant Professor of Clinical Pediatrics, Mount Sinai School of Medicine, and a practicing pediatrician in New York City.

Contents

Postpartum Program

This book will be your guide for one of the most important periods of your life and will enable you to remain healthy and physically fit throughout this challenging and exciting time. Divided into three sections, it is a complete program of proven and effective exercises for the pregnant and postpartum woman, as well as for the new infant.

Pregnancy causes physical and emotional changes in a woman, and the exercises in the pregnancy section have been specifically designed to deal with these unique changes. The instructions and routines have been carefully worked out so that in most cases you will be able to continue to exercise well into your ninth month.

The exercises are easy to perform, and the results will be apparent after several weeks. Besides keeping your body well toned, they will maintain high levels of energy. Keep in mind that it is important that you do the exercises regularly—consistency offers the most enduring and beneficial results.

After you have given birth, you will be eager to get back into shape and will want to begin the postpartum program. If you did not exercise regularly during your pregnancy, it will take you somewhat longer to regain your prepregnancy figure—but you will! And that is what's important.

The postpartum exercises deal mainly with those areas of the body that have been stretched out of their normal shape for months. These exercises help tone, trim, and reduce the stomach, hips and thighs, the waist and midriff area, and help strengthen the pectorals. These same exercises have a revitalizing effect and help dispel what is commonly known as postpartum blues.

The third section of the book is a series of starter exercises for the mother—or father—to do with the baby. Exercise sessions with your baby will prove to be rewarding times for you and your new infant—times of closeness, warmth, and affection. Your baby will feel the love and care of mommy and daddy and will benefit, of course, from the actual physical aspects of the exercises.

Infant exercises accelerate motor development, coordination, and agility. When exercise is a part of your infant's daily routine, your baby is more likely to sleep soundly, eat regularly, and be more relaxed than infants who are not exercised.

Altogether, this book will make your pregnancy and postpartum period comfortable and easy. You will be healthy and fit and your infant will get a great head start.

Pregnancy Program

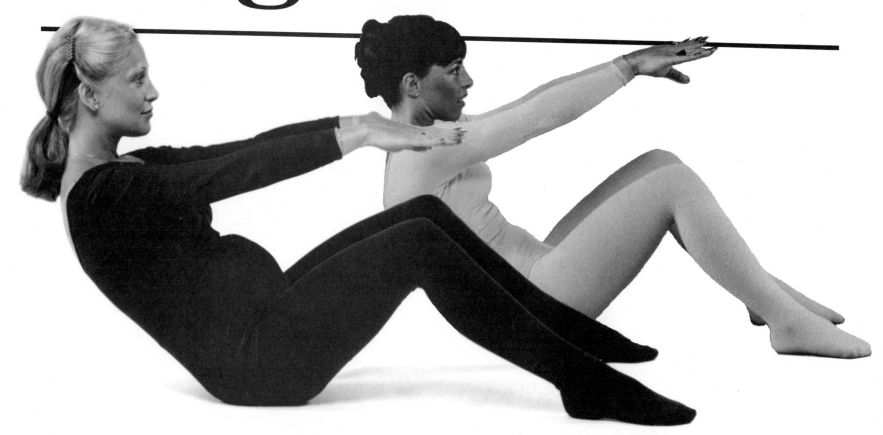

Pregnancy for the physically unfit can be an exhausting and unhappy experience. A pregnant woman should try to be in the best physical condition possible. After all, she is eating for two, breathing for two, and generating new cells for her own body as well as for the baby growing inside her; she is carrying around extra baggage that cannot be put aside even for a few minutes. It is there for nine months without respite. Indeed, as the pregnancy develops the burden will increase in size and weight, demanding ever larger quantities of oxygen and vital nutrients.

As a pregnant woman, you want to be as active and vigorous as you were before your pregnancy. To do so, you must get enough rest, eat properly, and stay physically fit. In addition to feeling good and looking good, being physically fit can make a difference between an easy or difficult labor and delivery. A woman who is weak and flabby will have less control over her muscles and less cardio-vascular endurance than a woman who has steadily and purposefully prepared her body.

What follows is an exercise program specially designed for the pregnant woman. Though nearly all obstetricians and gynecologists recommend an exercise program throughout pregnancy, you should not begin a fitness program until you have had a complete medical examination. You should have your doctor's explicit permission to undertake an exercise program. All the routines in this section have been carefully worked out for each stage of your pregnancy; they range from simple to moderately difficult. You should be able to do all of them, unless your doctor advises you against specific ones. They are divided into sections for different parts of the body and also into sections on breathing for relaxation, stretching to avoid cramps and spasms, and flexibility exercises so that your everyday movements do not become unnecessarily circumscribed.

Perhaps the least understood pregnancy exercises are those that strengthen the pelvic area. It is just above the pelvis that a new life is forming, and it is through the pelvis that this life will make its entrance into the world.

During pregnancy, the uterus presses down on the pelvic floor, which must be extremely strong to support the weight of the baby. And since the baby will pass through an opening of the pelvic floor at birth, the floor must also be extremely flexible—capable of stretching considerably, then returning to its original position. If you do all the pelvic exercises, you will be able to provide more support to the uterus before delivery and more assistance during the actual delivery. And since a sphincter in the pelvic floor controls elimination, a strong pelvis means good sphincter control, not only during pregnancy but afterward as well.

The pelvic floor is bordered by the abdominal wall, which also stretches during pregnancy. While the pelvic floor is severely stretched for a comparatively short period of time, the abdominal wall continues to expand continually for nine months. It must have elasticity to return to its original size and shape. If you have weak abdominal muscles, your growing stomach will put a strain on your lower back that can result in severe and debilitating pain. Therefore, a number of effective lower back and stomach exercises are included in this book.

The leg exercises serve several purposes. They will ease or prevent muscle spasms and cramps in your calves and in the backs of your thighs. They will also stretch the insides of the thighs, an area where the muscles must stretch significantly during delivery. And finally, the exercises will enhance the efficiency of your circulatory system, diminishing your chances of developing varicose veins and hemorrhoids, two unfortunately common afflictions associated with pregnancy.

As your pregnancy advances, the size and weight of your breasts will increase naturally, thus it is important to have strong pectoral muscles that will provide support. The arm exercises will strengthen these muscles and help reduce tension in the upper back area. It is advisable, whether you are large-breasted or not, to wear a bra during your pregnancy—certainly whenever you exercise.

The complete fitness program that follows will not

only keep your muscles toned, strong, and flexible, but it will also have a positive effect on your entire circulatory system. While you are pregnant, your body has from 20 to 40 percent more blood than normally. Exercise will keep blood vessels strong and flexible and aid circulation.

As a regular fitness program can make a nonpregnant woman feel vigorous, strong, and healthy, so a pregnant woman can feel good about herself. A fit pregnant woman will also suffer less from fatigue and its complement, irritability. Indeed, exercise is a tonic: done regularly, it will give you the energy, the will, and the spirit to enjoy all the marvelous, life-enhancing aspects of pregnancy and childbirth.

General rules you should follow:

- Have a complete physical examination and get your doctor's explicit permission to undertake an exercise program.
- Never overdo. Never push yourself beyond your threshold of comfortable endurance. If a particular exercise causes pain, stop immediately.
- Exercise in short but regular sessions, perhaps 4 times a day, for 5 to 10 minutes each time.
- Make sure you follow each step of an exercise and do not rush to complete it.
- Breathe regularly while exercising. Never hold your breath; never exhale and forget to take another breath of air.
- Never exercise when you feel nausea, dizzy, or ill in any way. If you do, consult your doctor.
- Do recumbent exercises on a cushiony towel, blanket, or mat.
- Exercise to upbeat music and, if possible, in the company of other pregnant women.
- There are exercises for all sections of your body; do not concentrate on any one section and ignore the others.

Supine Pelvic Floor Isometric

The pelvic area should be strong and flexible. The contractions in this exercise help to strengthen this important region.

Suzy's Program

First through ninth month:
repeat sequence 3 times, and whenever you have time

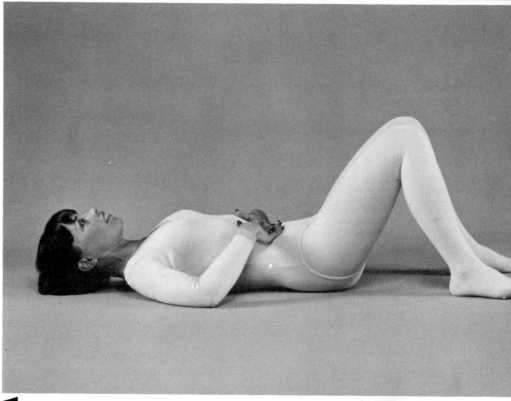

1

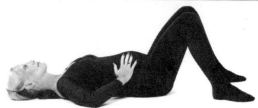

Lie on your back with your knees bent and about 12 inches apart. Keep the soles of your feet flat on the floor and place the palms of your hands on your stomach. Your lower back should be pressed against the floor.

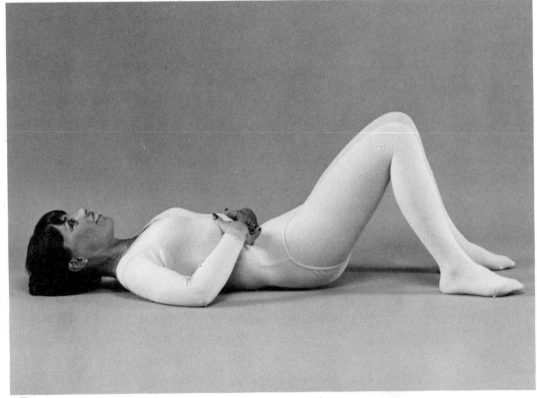

2

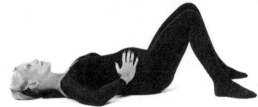

Contract and tighten your stomach and fanny muscles. You will feel your stomach muscles tighten beneath your fingers. The lower half of your fanny should lift slightly off the floor. Hold for 4 seconds, then relax.

Praying Pelvis

This exercise not only tightens and strengthens the pelvic area, but it also strengthens the stomach muscles, lower back, and thighs.

Suzy's Program

First through third month: repeat sequence 8 times

Fourth through sixth month: repeat sequence 12 times

Seventh through ninth month: repeat sequence 6 times

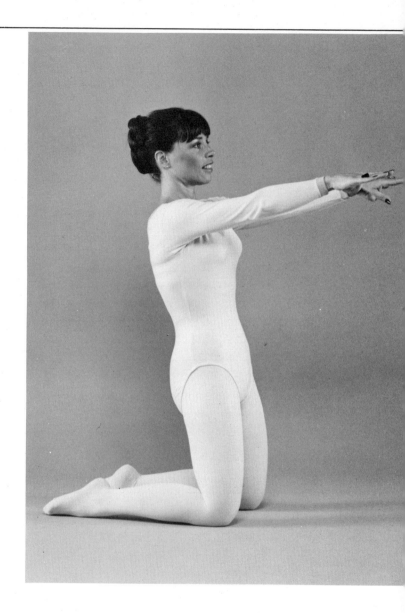

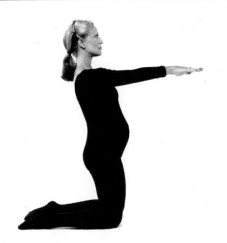

1

Kneel with your knees about 12 inches apart, keeping your torso straight and your insteps flat on the floor. Stretch your arms straight out so that they are parallel to the floor.

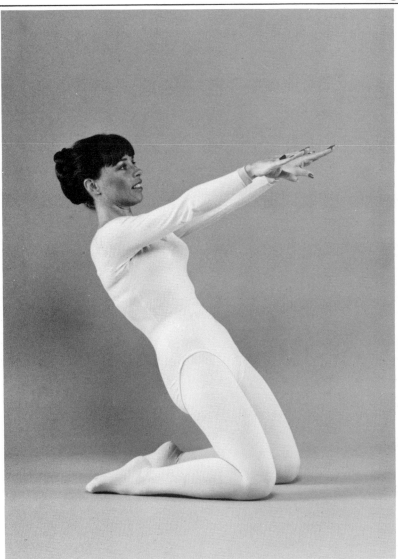

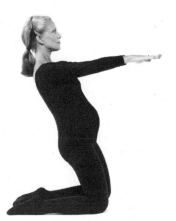

2

Tighten and contract your stomach and fanny muscles. Lean back slightly, keeping your body from your shoulders to your knees as straight as possible. Hold for 4 seconds, then return to the original position.

Kneeling Pelvic Tilt

This is a particularly effective exercise to strengthen the stomach and lower back muscles. It is also good for toning the upper thighs.

Suzy's Program

First through third month: repeat sequence 8 times

Fourth through sixth month: repeat sequence 16 times

Seventh through ninth month: repeat sequence 8 times

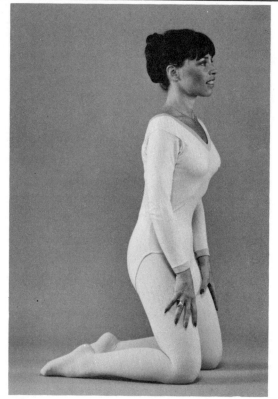
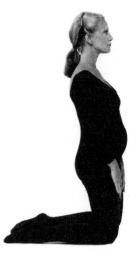

1

Kneel with your knees about 12 inches apart, keeping your torso straight and your insteps flat on the floor. Place your hands on your thighs.

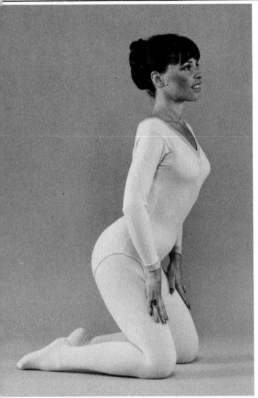
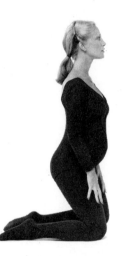

2

Arch your lower back and stick out your fanny.

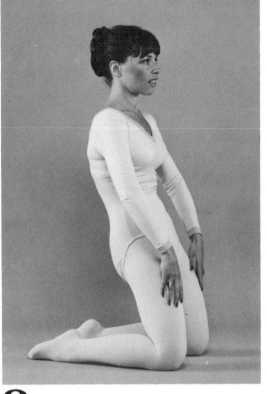
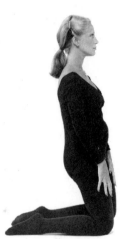

3

Tuck your fanny under, pushing your pelvis forward and upward. Do not move your shoulders.

The Pelvic Tilt

This superb exercise strengthens the entire pelvic area so that you can lift and tuck your pelvis without strain during delivery.

Suzy's Program

First through third month: repeat sequence 8 times

Fourth through sixth month: repeat sequence 16 times

Seventh through ninth month: repeat sequence 8 times

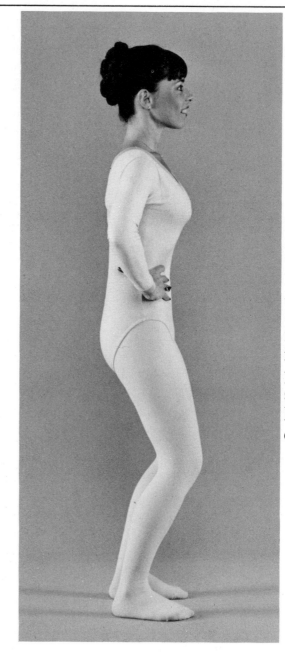

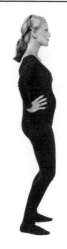

1

Stand with your feet about 12 inches apart and your knees slightly bent. Place your hands on your waist.

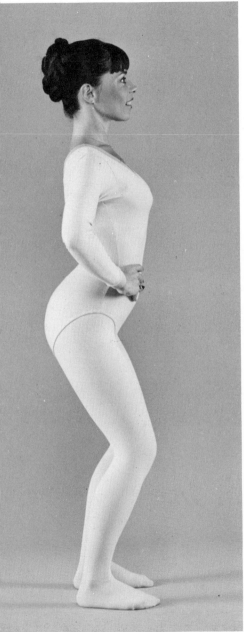

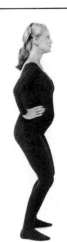

2

Arch your lower
back and stick
out your fanny.

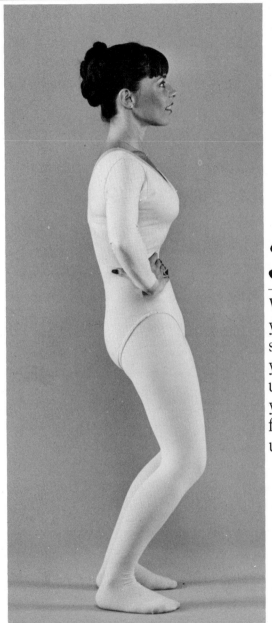

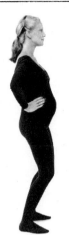

3

Without moving
your knees or
shoulders, tuck
your fanny
under, pushing
your pelvis
forward and
upward.

The Pelvic Circle

This exercise strengthens muscles on all sides of the pelvic area. Such muscular control will not only be an additional aid during delivery, but the strengthened muscles will help you regain your waistline during the postpartum period.

Suzy's Program

First through third month: repeat sequence 4 times

Fourth through sixth month: repeat sequence 8 times

Seventh through ninth month: repeat sequence 4 times

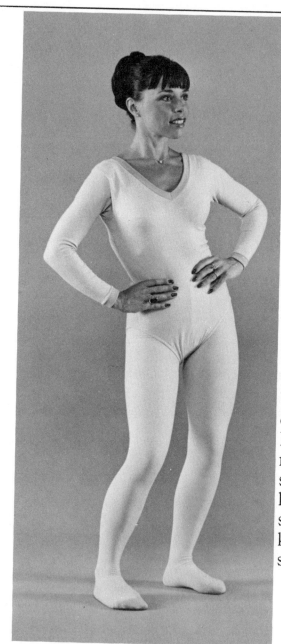
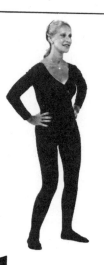

1

Stand with your feet about 12 inches apart, knees slightly bent and hands on your waist. Begin your rotation by sticking your left hip out to the side. Keep your knees and shoulders still.

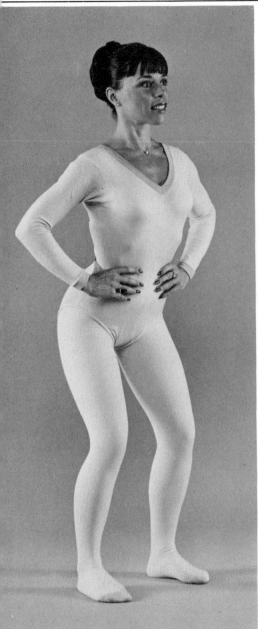

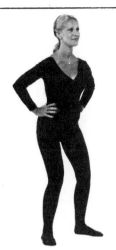

2

Continue to
rotate your pelvic
area. Arch
your lower back
and stick out
your fanny.

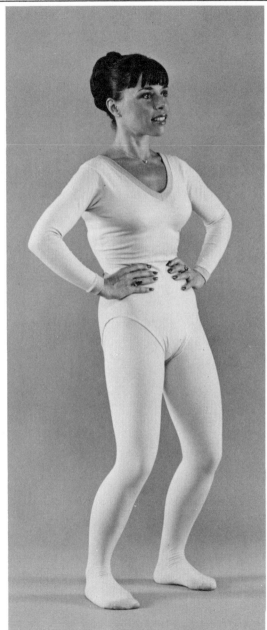

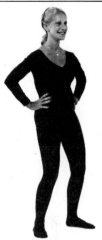

3

Rotate your
pelvic area to
the right; then
tuck your pelvis
under. Repeat
the rotation in
the opposite
direction.

Modified Sit-up

Before beginning this exercise, make sure your legs are far enough apart so that your stomach does not collide with your upper legs. If you cannot do the complete sit-up, start in a sitting position and slowly lower your torso to the count of 4.

Suzy's Program

First through third month: repeat sequence 8 times

Fourth through sixth month: repeat sequence 16 times

Seventh through ninth month: repeat sequence 8 times

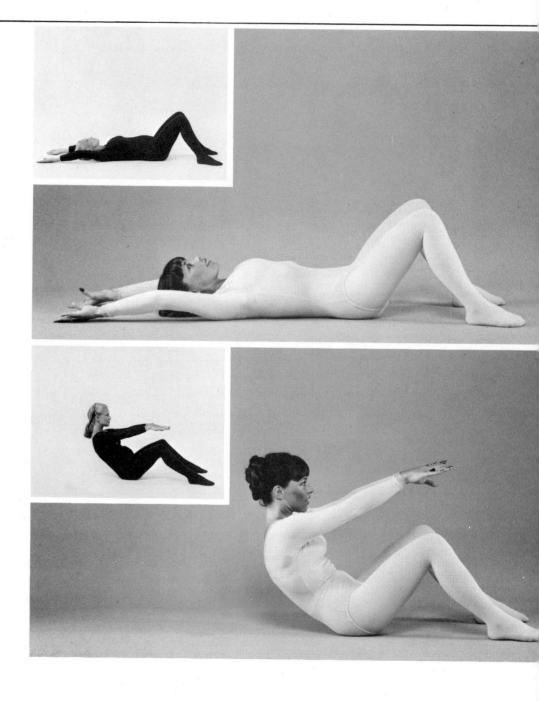

1

Lie on your back with knees bent and feet flat on the floor. Your legs and knees should be about 12 inches apart and your arms outstretched on the floor above your head.

2

In one graceful movement, swing your arms up and forward, while bringing your torso into a sitting position with your back rounded.

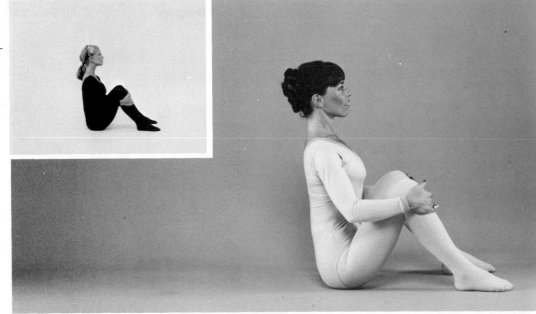

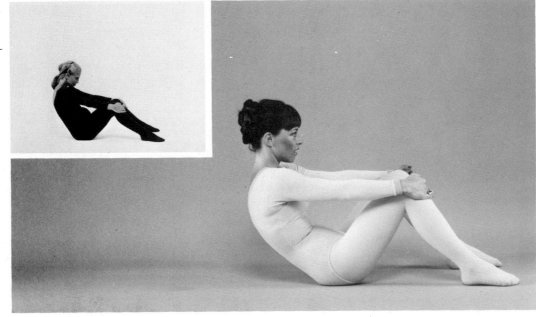

3

Clasp your knees with your hands and straighten your back. Hold this position for 4 seconds. Be sure not to tighten your shoulders.

4

Round your back and slowly lower your torso to the original position with your back flat on the floor.

31

Supine Crossover

The customary stomach exercises strengthen muscles by either vertical or horizontal contractions. In this exercise, however, the front as well as the sides of the stomach are strengthened by the crossover movements.

Suzy's Program

First through third month: repeat sequence 4 times

Fourth through sixth month: repeat sequence 8 times

Seventh through ninth month: repeat sequence 4 times

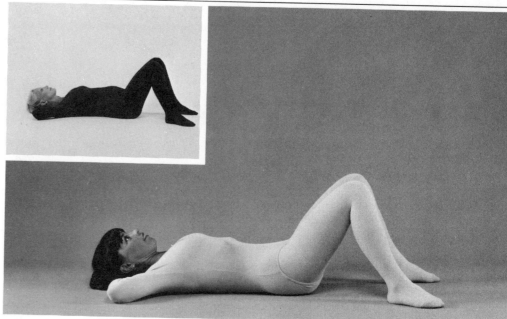

1

Lie on your back with knees bent and feet flat on the floor. Your legs and knees should be about 12 inches apart. Clasp your hands behind your neck.

2

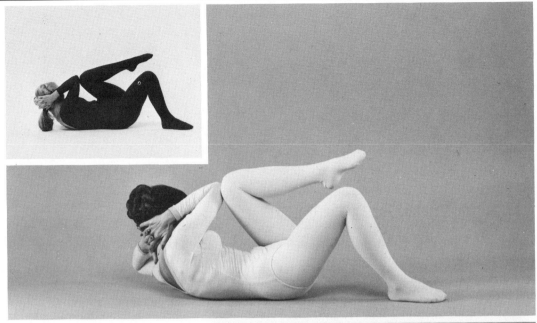

Lift your head and right shoulder off the floor. At the same time, raise your left leg and touch your right elbow to your left knee. Keep your toes pointed.

3

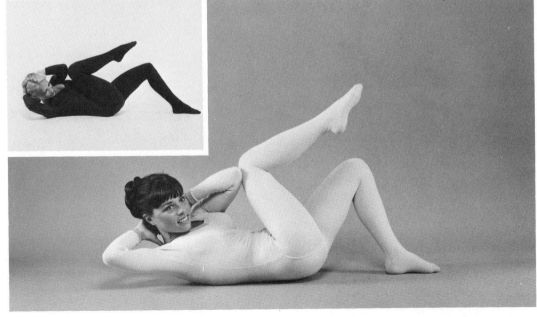

Return to the original position and reverse the crossover.

Crossover Sit-up

This exercise combines the best aspects of the previous two exercises. If you find that your stomach begins to get in the way, just twist your body as you get up. It will not be necessary to touch your elbows to your knees. If you experience any lower back pain while doing this exercise, consult your doctor.

Suzy's Program

First through third month: repeat sequence 4 times

Fourth through sixth month: repeat sequence 8 times

Seventh through ninth month: repeat sequence 4 times

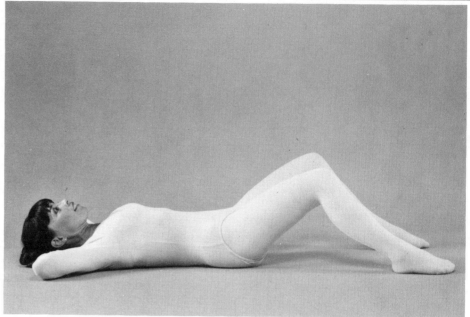

1

Lie on your back with knees bent and feet flat on the floor. Your legs and knees should be about 12 inches apart to allow room for your baby. Clasp your hands behind your neck.

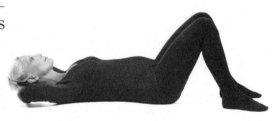

34

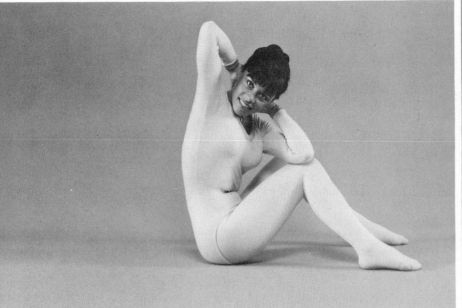

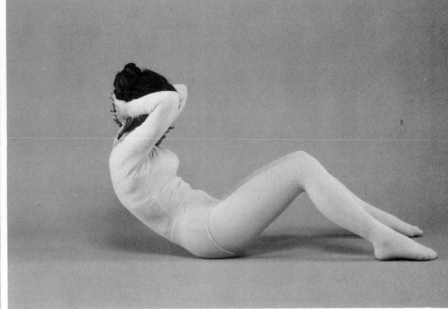

2

With your hands clasped
behind your neck and your
feet flat on the floor, sit up
and twist your torso,
touching your left elbow
to your right knee.

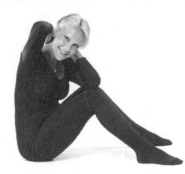

3

Roll down to a count of 4 and
press your lower back
against the floor. Repeat,
twisting to the left and
touching your right elbow
to your left knee.

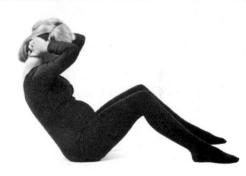

On-elbows Bicycle

This is an extremely effective exercise for strengthening the stomach as well as the lower back. After completing 8 pedaling motions with each leg, lean onto the right side of your fanny and pedal 8 times. Then lean onto the left side, and pedal 8 times more. Be sure to keep your stomach muscles tightened throughout the exercise.

Suzy's Program

First through ninth month: complete sequence at least once a day

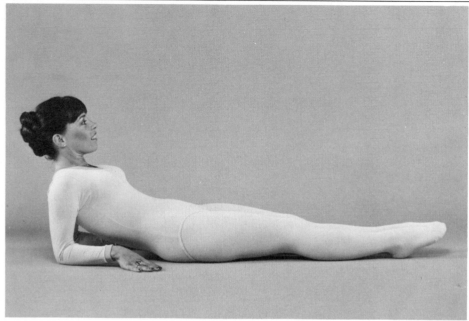

1

Lie on the floor with your torso propped up on your elbows. Your legs should be straight, feet together and pointed. Your forearms should be parallel to your body. Keep the palms of your hands flat on the floor.

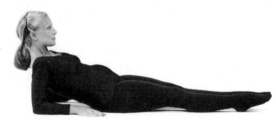

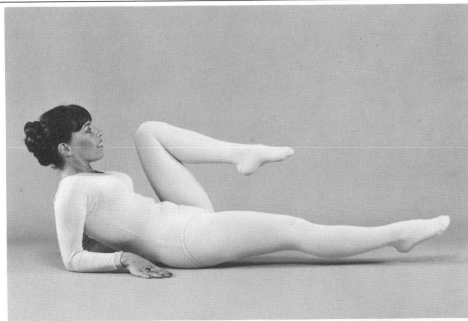

2

Begin to bicycle by bringing your left knee to your chest. Then, as you straighten and lower your leg to within 6 inches of the floor, bend your right knee to your chest.

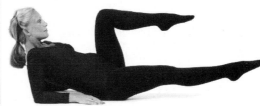

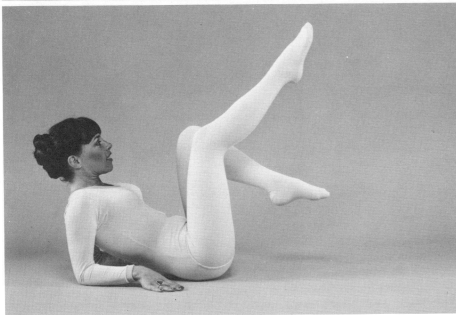

3

Continue this alternating movement, making 8 pedaling motions with each leg. Then lean onto first one side of your fanny and then the other, making 8 more pedaling motions on each side.

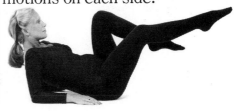

Round and Straighten

Do not tense or tighten your shoulders during this simple and pleasant stomach exercise. Be sure your legs are far enough apart to allow room for your growing stomach.

Suzy's Program

First through third month: repeat sequence 8 times

Fourth through sixth month: repeat sequence 16 times

Seventh through ninth month: repeat sequence 8 times

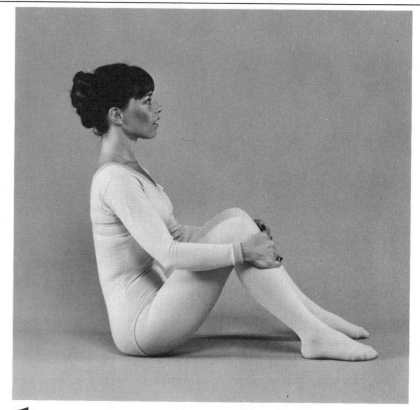

1

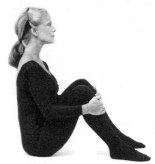

Sit with your knees bent, feet flat on the floor and hands clasped below your knees. Your knees and feet should be about 12 inches apart.

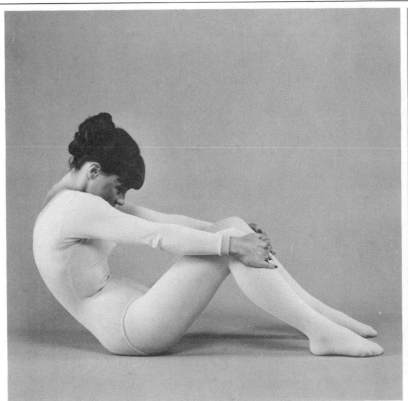

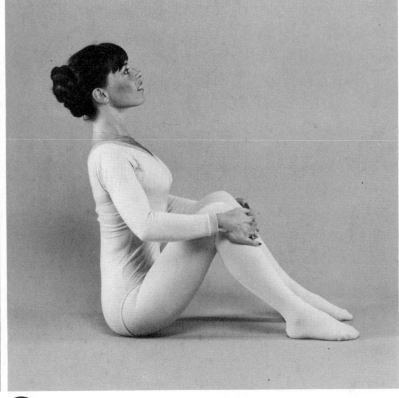

2

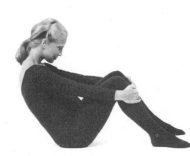

Round your back and bring your shoulders forward, straightening your arms. Let your head drop to your chest. Keep your feet flat on the floor. Tighten your stomach muscles and hold this position for 4 seconds.

3

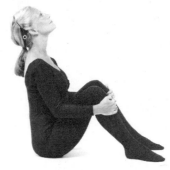

Slowly straighten your torso by pushing from your lower back and bending your arms. Tighten your stomach muscles and look up. Hold this position for 4 seconds.

The Kitty Stretch

This exercise strengthens both the lower and upper back areas. It is especially effective in reducing muscular tension in the back and shoulder regions.

Suzy's Program

First through third month: repeat sequence 6 times

Fourth through sixth month: repeat sequence 8 times

Seventh through ninth month: repeat sequence 4 times

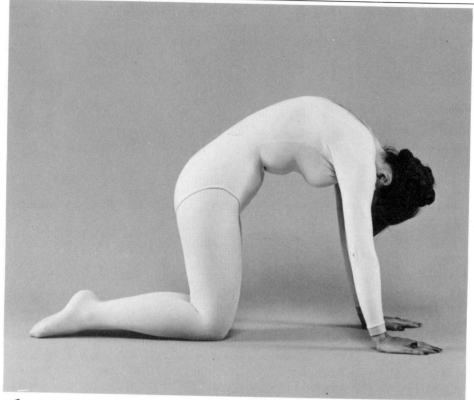

1

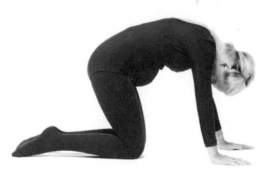

Beginning on your hands and knees, round your upper back and lower your head, stretching out the back of your neck. Tighten your stomach muscles. Hold this position for 4 seconds.

40

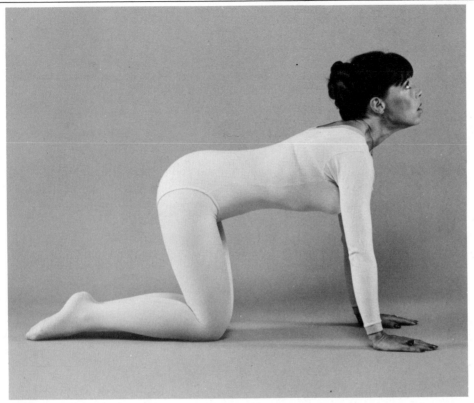

2

In one continuous motion, lift your head, stretching out the front of your neck, and flattening your upper back. Allow your lower back to sag slightly. Never force your lower back to sag farther than it will comfortably go.

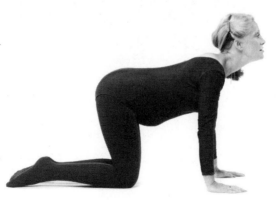

Back Flat, Leg Lower

This is one of the most effective lower back exercises, but it must be done properly. When you lower your legs, do not let your lower back lift off the floor; if it does, you have gone too far and may hurt yourself.

Suzy's Program

First through third month: repeat sequence 4 times

Fourth through sixth month: repeat sequence 8 times

Seventh through ninth month: repeat sequence 4 times

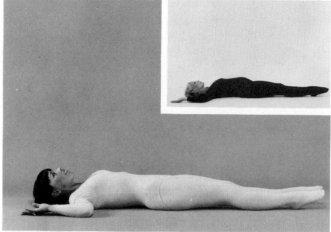

1

Lie on your back, legs straight and feet pointed, with your forearms on the floor parallel to your head.

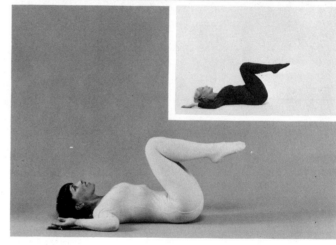

2

Bend your legs and bring them over your chest.

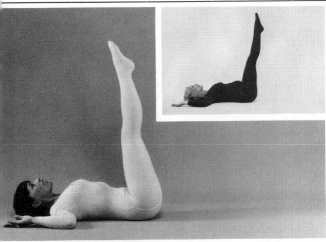

3

Straighten your legs so that they are perpendicular to the floor. Keep your legs together, feet pointed, and press your lower back against the floor.

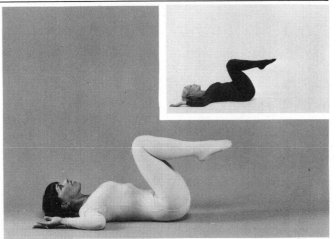

4

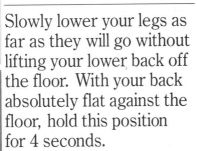

Slowly lower your legs as far as they will go without lifting your lower back off the floor. With your back absolutely flat against the floor, hold this position for 4 seconds.

5

Bring your knees over your chest and rest for 4 seconds. After the final series, bring your knees over your chest and slowly lower your feet to the floor. Never lower straightened legs to the floor. If you do, you might strain your lower back.

The Bent-leg Twist

Lower back pain and fatigue are common complaints during pregnancy. This exercise is one of the great tension relievers for lower backs, and it is strongly recommended. Try to keep your legs together.

Suzy's Program

First through third month: repeat sequence 12 times

Fourth through sixth month: repeat sequence 16 times

Seventh through ninth month: repeat sequence 12 times

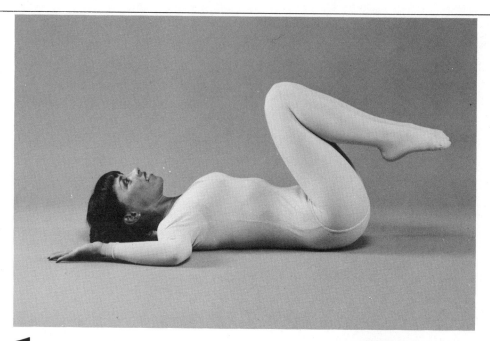

1

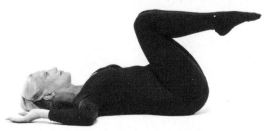

Lie on your back with your knees bent over your torso, feet pointed, and your forearms parallel to your head.

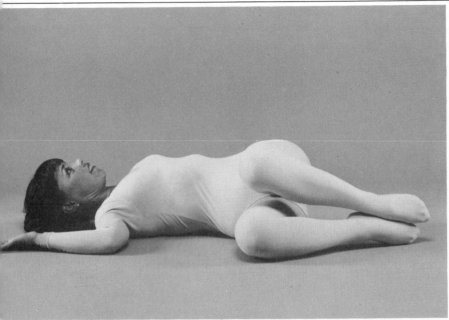

2

Twisting to the right from your waist, lower your bent legs to the floor. Be sure to keep your shoulders flat on the floor.

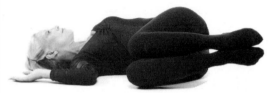

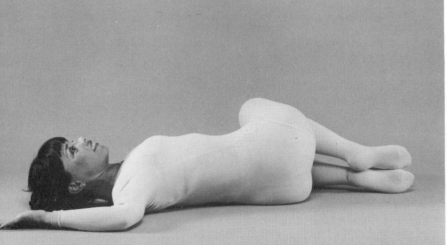

3

Keeping your legs bent and together, bring them up over your torso, then twist to the left and lower your legs to floor.

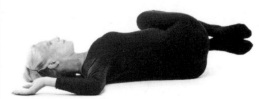

Arch and Flatten

This simple but effective exercise strengthens the lower back muscles and lessens the strain in the lower back region throughout, as well as after, your pregnancy.

Suzy's Program

First through third month: repeat sequence 8 times, once a day

Fourth through sixth month: repeat sequence 8 times, twice a day

Seventh through ninth month: repeat sequence 8 times, three times a day, and whenever experiencing pain

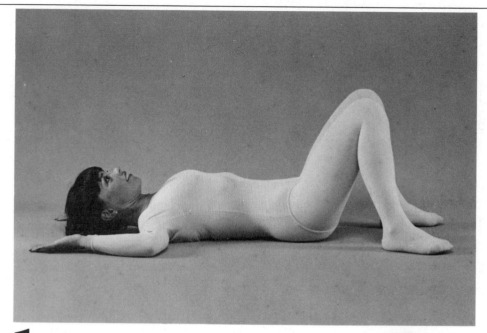

1

Lie on your back with your knees bent and feet flat on the floor. Your knees and feet should be about 12 inches apart. Place your forearms on the floor parallel to your head.

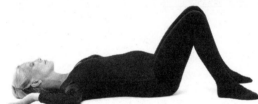

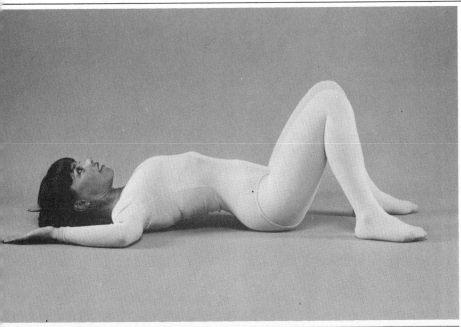

2

Arch your lower back so that it is about 2 inches off the floor. Be sure your upper back and fanny remain on the floor. Hold this position for 2 seconds.

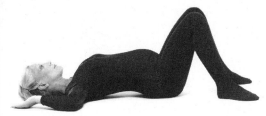

3

Tuck your pelvis under so that your lower back is pressed flat against the floor. Hold this position for 4 seconds, then relax.

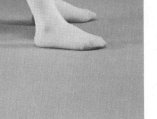

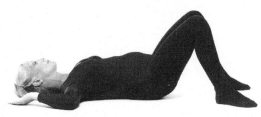

Sitting Arch and Flatten

One of the advantages of this exercise is that it can be done just about anywhere you are sitting. It relieves tensions that are common and alleviates the strain on the lower back.

Suzy's Program

First through third month: repeat sequence 16 times

Fourth through sixth month: repeat sequence 24 times

Seventh through ninth month: repeat sequence 16 times

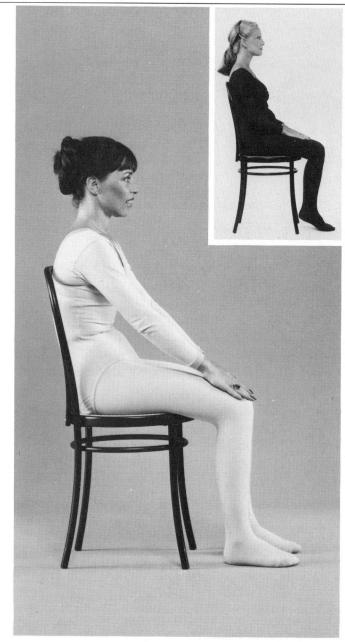

1

Sit on a chair that has a straight back. Press your lower back against the back of the chair and hold this position for 4 seconds.

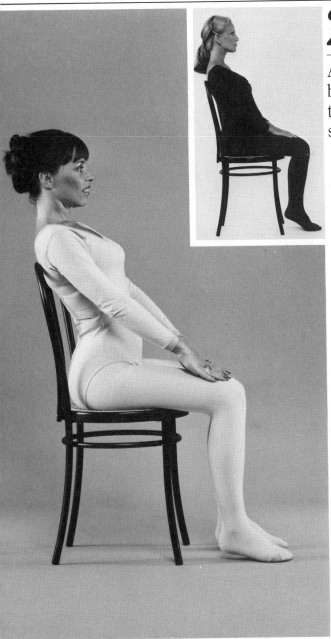

2

Arch your lower back and hold this position for 2 seconds.

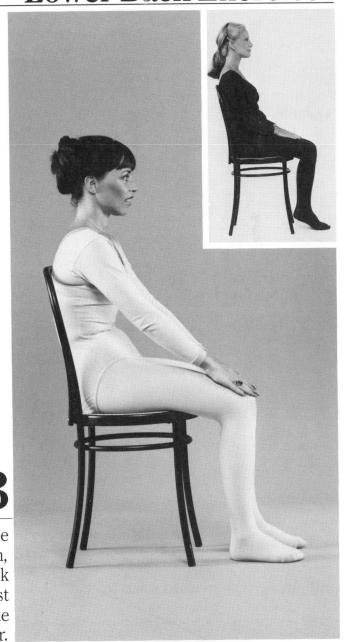

3

Return to the original position, your lower back pressed against the back of the chair.

Skydiving

This simple exercise helps to strengthen your pectoral muscles, which provide essential support to your breasts, especially during pregnancy.

Suzy's Program

First through third month: repeat sequence 6 times

Fourth through sixth month: repeat sequence 8 times

Seventh through ninth month: repeat sequence 12 times

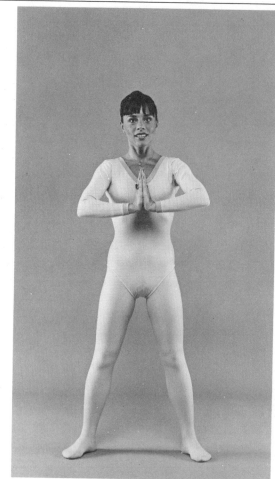

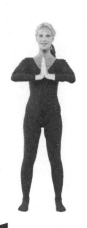

1

Stand straight, with your feet apart and your palms pressed together in front of your chest.

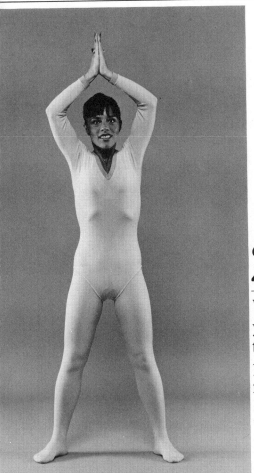

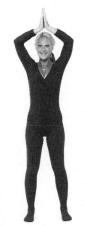

2

While pressing your palms together, tighten your pectoral muscles and slowly raise your hands over your head. Hold for 4 seconds.

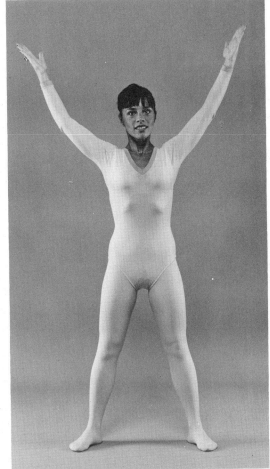

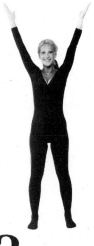

3

Release your hands, stretching your arms to form a "V" above your head.

Airplane Stretch

An easy exercise that keeps your pectoral muscles strong as it strengthens and straightens your upper back so that pendulous breasts do not put unnecessary strain on your posture.

Suzy's Program

First through third month: repeat sequence 12 times

Fourth through sixth month: repeat sequence 24 times

Seventh through ninth month: repeat sequence 12 times

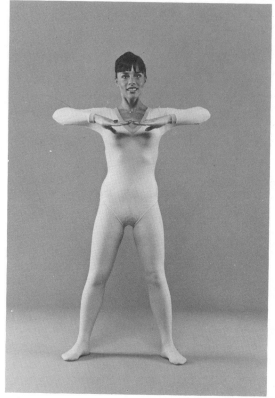 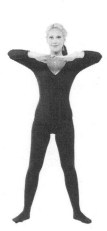

1

Stand straight with your feet apart and bend your arms at shoulder level so that your fingers touch in front of your chest.

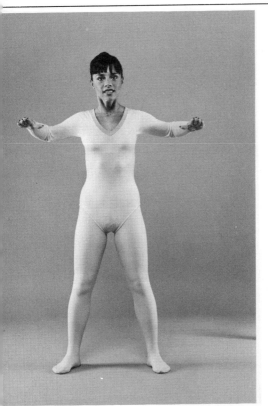

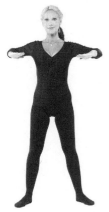

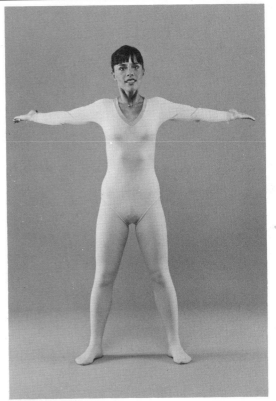

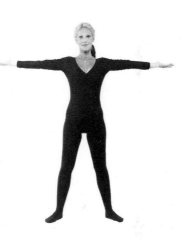

2

Swiftly, but gently, move your arms back as far as is comfortably possible, keeping them bent so your elbows point behind. Return your arms to their original position in front of you.

3

Turn your palms up toward the ceiling, and swing your arms out and back, straightening your elbows. Your arms should be outstretched, palms up, at shoulder height. Return to the original position.

Butterfly Salute

While doing this graceful exercise, it is important that your bent elbows are pointed back rather than out to the side.

Suzy's Program

First through third month: repeat sequence 8 times with each arm, then 4 times with both arms together

Fourth through sixth month: repeat sequence 12 times with each arm, then 6 times with both arms together

Seventh through ninth month: repeat sequence 8 times with each arm, then 4 times with both arms together

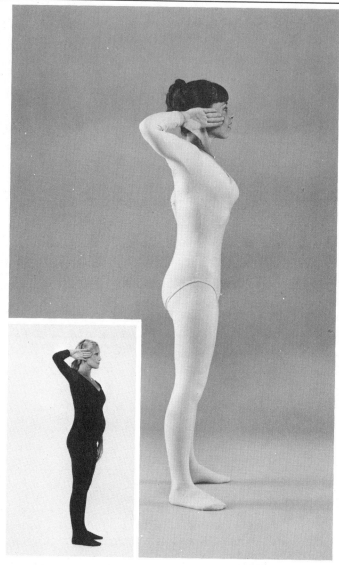

1

Stand straight with your feet apart and your right elbow up and back. Keep your right palm facing out, fingers against your cheek. Your left arm is relaxed at your side.

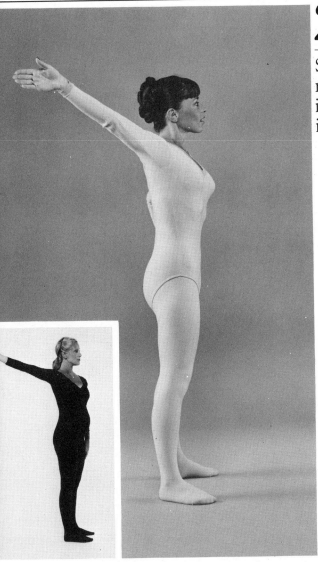

2

Straighten your right arm so that it swings up and in back of you.

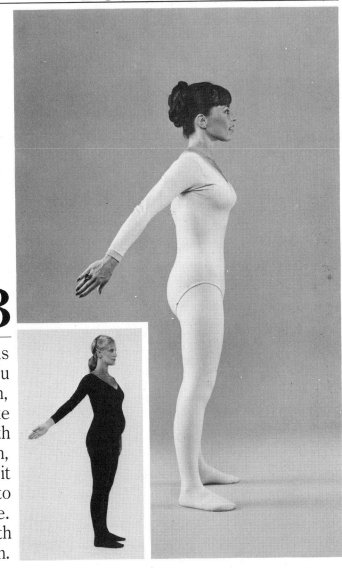

3

Reaching out as far as you comfortably can, continue to make a half-circle with your arm, bringing it downward to rest at your side. Repeat with your left arm.

Wall Push-up

This variation of the push-up strengthens your arms and shoulders as well as your pectoral muscles.

Suzy's Program

First through third month: repeat sequence 6 times

Fourth through sixth month: repeat sequence 8 times

Seventh through ninth month: repeat sequence 6 times

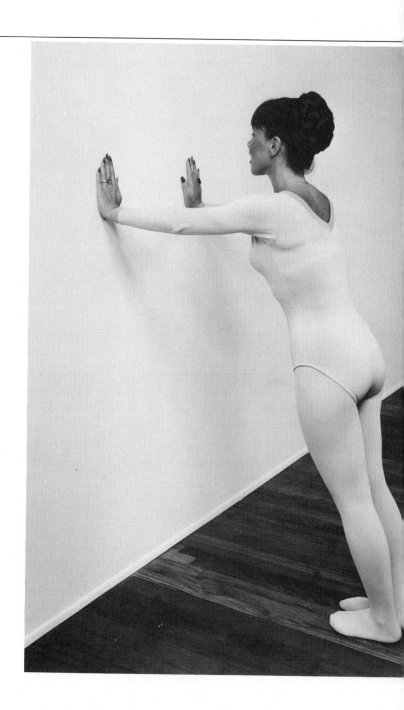

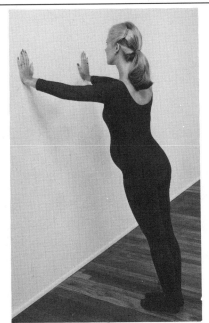

1

Standing with your legs together and about 2 feet from the wall, place your hands against the wall at shoulder height.

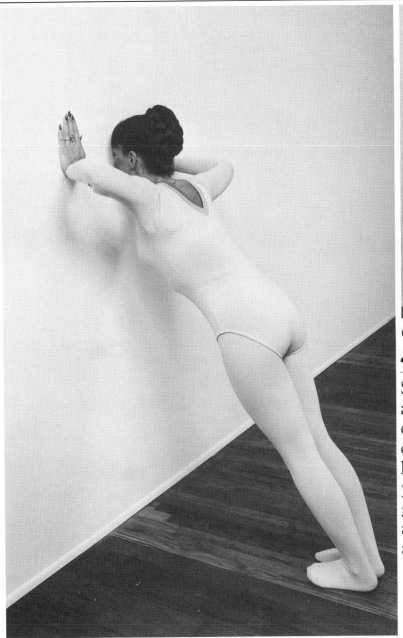

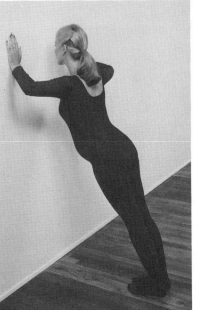

2

Slowly bend your elbows and bring your face as close to the wall as you can without lifting your heels off the floor. Keep your body straight. Then gently straighten your arms, pushing your body away from the wall.

Paint the Wall

Do this exercise slowly and cautiously. From your seventh month on, be especially careful not to put pressure on your stomach.

Suzy's program

First through third month: complete sequence once

Fourth through sixth month: repeat sequence twice

Seventh through ninth month: complete sequence once

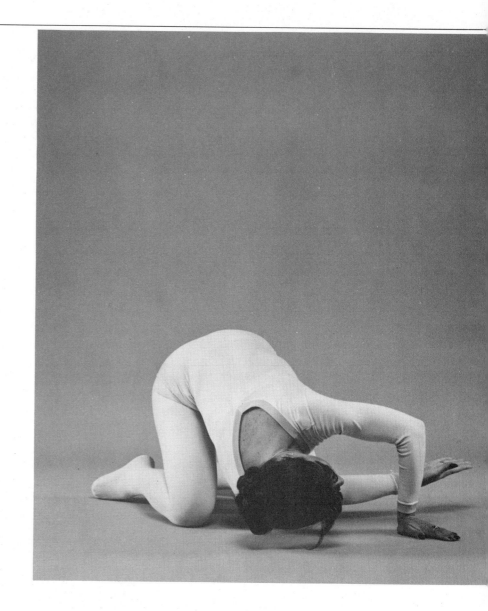

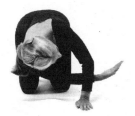

1

Starting on your hands and knees, bend your left elbow and stretch your right hand under your left side as far as you comfortably can.

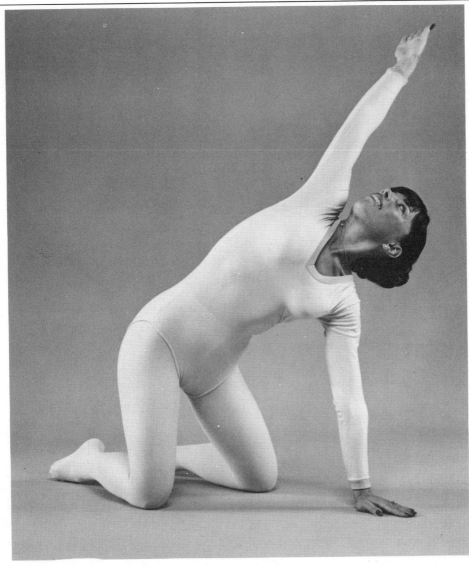

2

Straighten your left arm and swing your right arm up, stretching it as far as possible. Turn your head to look at your raised fingers. Swing and straighten your arm 6 times. Repeat with your left arm.

Standing "C"

To do this exercise correctly, stretch your arms while you bounce. You should feel your muscles stretch along your waist and ribs.

Suzy's Program

First through third month: repeat sequence 4 times

Fourth through sixth month: repeat sequence 8 times

Seventh through ninth month: repeat sequence 6 times

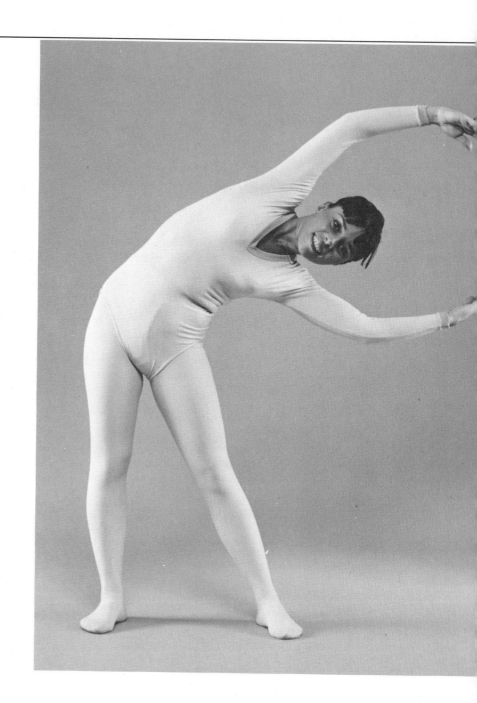

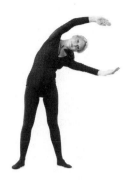

1

Stand straight
with your feet
apart and
stretch your
arms over your
head so that
your fingers
point at one
another. Curve
your torso as far
to the right as
you can without
bending forward
or arching your
back. Gently
bounce to the
right 4 times.

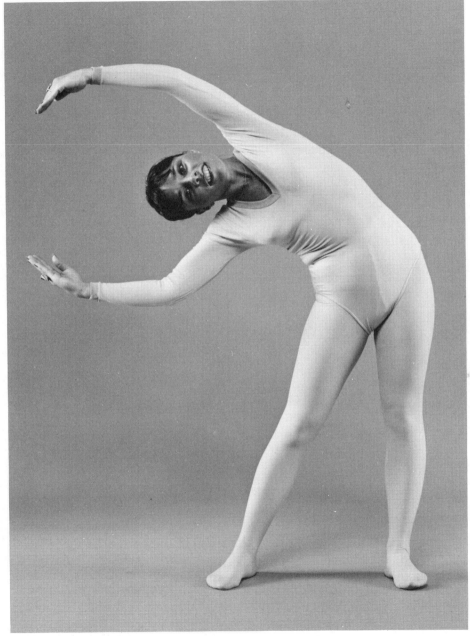

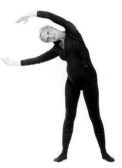

2

Curve your
torso to the left
and gently
bounce 4 times
to the left.

Swing High, Swing Low

When you do this exercise correctly, you can feel the muscles stretch along your waist and ribs. Do not lean forward or arch your back. Keep your hips facing forward.

Suzy's Program

First through third month: repeat sequence 8 times

Fourth through sixth month: repeat sequence 16 times

Seventh through ninth month: repeat sequence 8 times

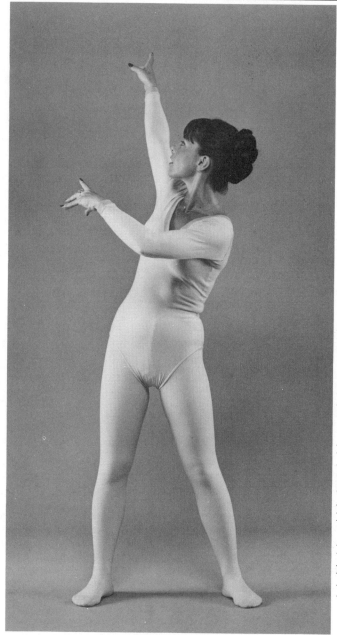

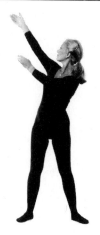

1

Stand straight with your feet apart. Swing your arms to the right so that your right arm is straight and raised behind you and your left arm is bent in front of you. Your head should follow the movement of your right arm.

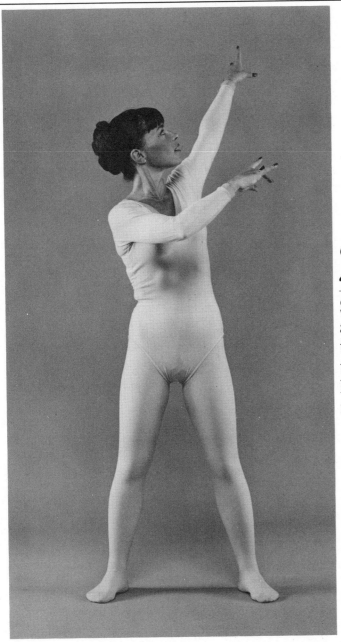

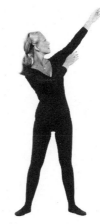

2

Swing your arms
and upper torso
to the left,
turning your
head to face your
raised left arm.

Stretch and Twist

It is important in this exercise to stretch with your arms as far as you comfortably can, keeping both your arms and legs straight.

Suzy's Program

First through third month: repeat sequence 8 times

Fourth through sixth month: repeat sequence 6 times

Seventh through ninth month: repeat sequence 4 times

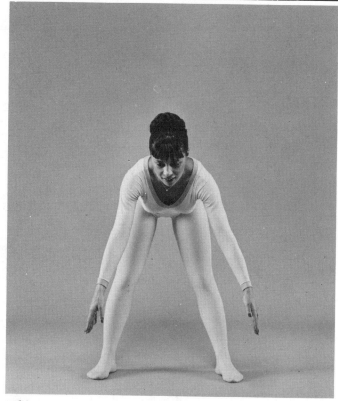

1

Standing with your legs straight and feet apart, bend forward at the hips so that your torso is parallel to the floor. Your arms should be stretched toward the floor.

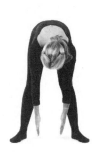

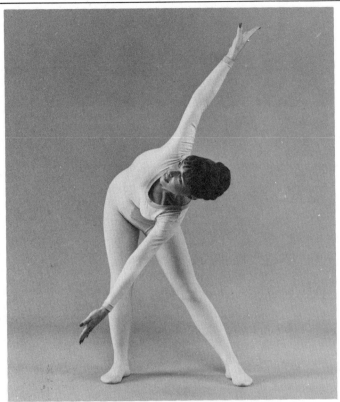

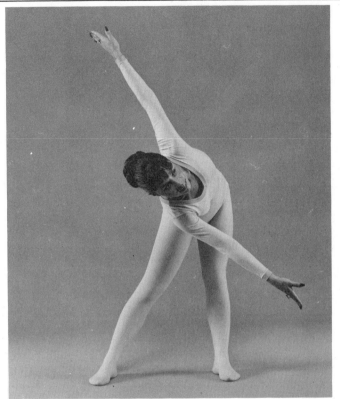

2

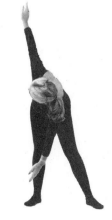

Turn your torso and head to the right so that your right arm is raised and your left arm is in front of your right leg.

3

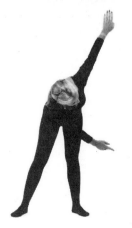

In the same manner, turn your torso and head to the left so that your left arm is raised and your right arm is in front of your left leg.

Taking Off

This is one of the most effective exercises for keeping upper arms toned and flexible. Be sure to keep the circular motions of your arms small and smooth.

Suzy's Program

First through third month: complete sequence once

Fourth through sixth month: repeat sequence twice

Seventh through ninth month: complete sequence once

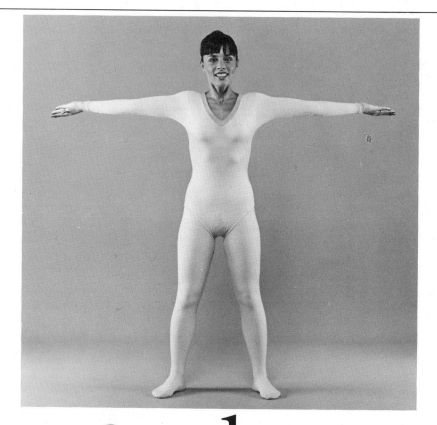

1

Stand straight, with your feet apart and arms stretched out to the sides at shoulder height. Turn the palms of both hands up, then continue turning them until they are facing as far back as is comfortably possible.

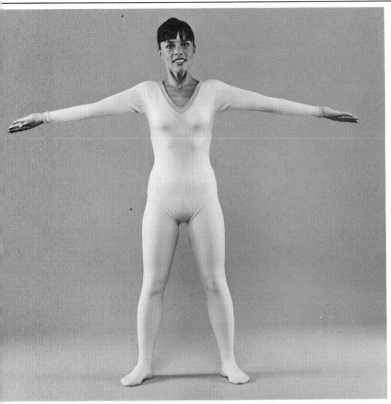

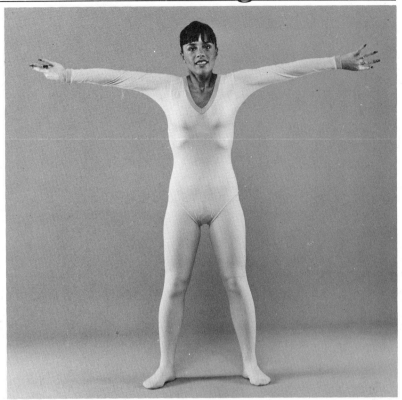

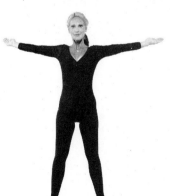

2

With your palms turned back, rotate your arms in a backward motion, making 8 small full circles. Keep your arms straight.

3

While keeping your arms stretched straight out to the side, turn your palms down, then back and up so they face the ceiling. Rotate your arms in a foward motion, making 8 small full circles.

Table Lift

In this exercise, keep your arms straight. Your body should form a straight line between your knees and shoulders when it is raised off the floor.

Suzy's Program

First through third month: repeat sequence 6 times

Fourth through sixth month: repeat sequence 12 times

Seventh through ninth month: repeat sequence 6 times

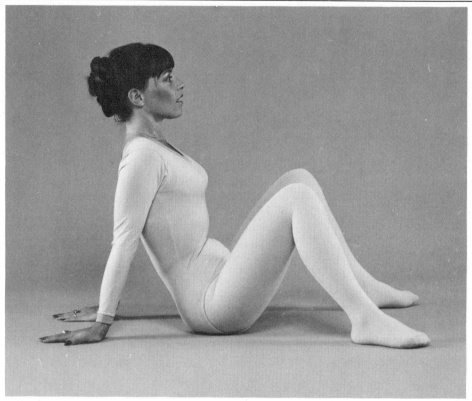

1

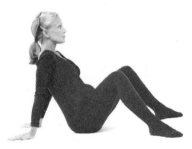

Sit on the floor with your legs slightly apart, knees bent, and feet flat on the floor. Place your palms several inches behind your fanny, fingers pointed away from your body.

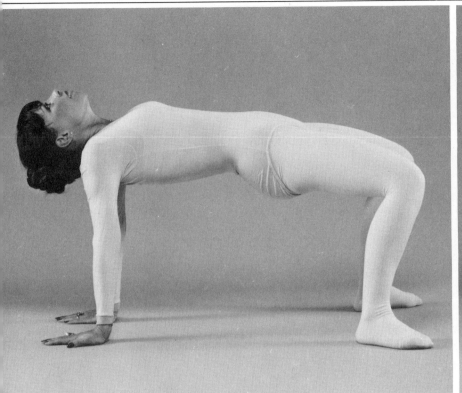

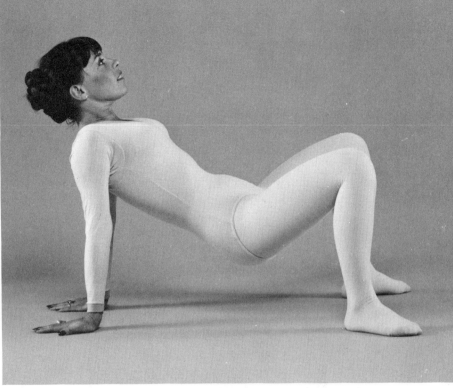

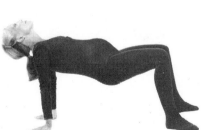

2

Lift your fanny and push your entire torso into the air so it is parallel to the floor. Do not bend at the waist. Hold the raised position for 6 seconds.

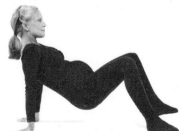

3

Slowly lower your fanny and return to the original position.

Supine Air Kick

It is important to keep your lower back flat on the floor during this exercise.

Suzy's Program

First through third month: complete sequence once

Fourth through six month: repeat sequence twice

Seventh through ninth month: complete sequence once

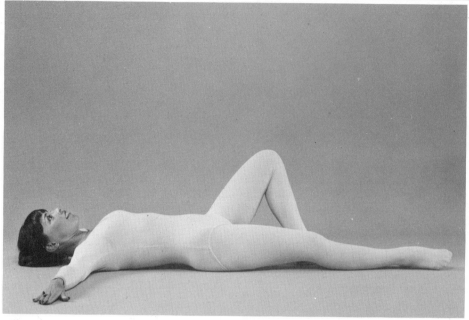

1

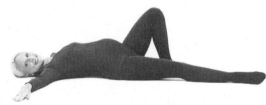

Lie on your back and stretch your arms straight out to the sides. Bend your left leg at the knee, keeping the sole of your left foot flat on the floor. Press your lower back against the floor. Turn your right knee out to the side.

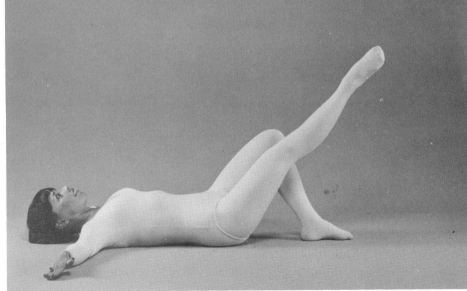

2

Without moving your left leg, lift your right leg until it is perpendicular to the floor. Keep your leg straight, turned out and foot pointed.

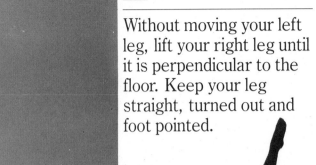

3

With your knee still turned out, slowly lower your right leg, keeping your back flat on the floor. Raise and lower your right leg 6 times, then repeat with your left leg.

Raised Side Scissors

In this exercise, keep both legs raised about 6 inches off the floor. Your legs should be stretched to make them as long as possible and your knees should face forward at all times.

Suzy's Program

First through third month: complete sequence once

Fourth through six month: repeat sequence twice

Seventh through ninth month: complete sequence once

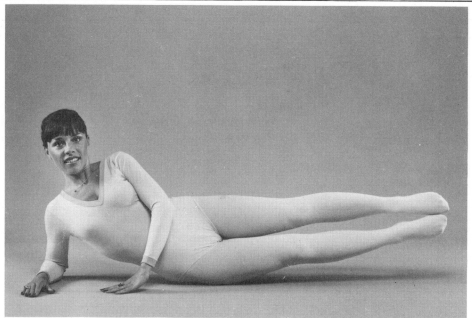

1

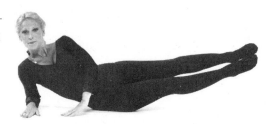

Lie on your right side with your torso propped up on your right elbow and forearm. Rest your left hand in front of you. Keep your legs straight with feet pointed and raised about 6 inches off the floor.

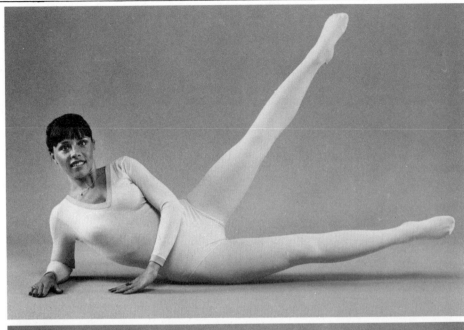

2

Raise and lower your left leg 8 times, keeping your right leg in the raised position.

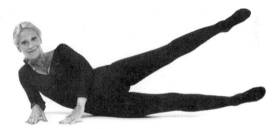

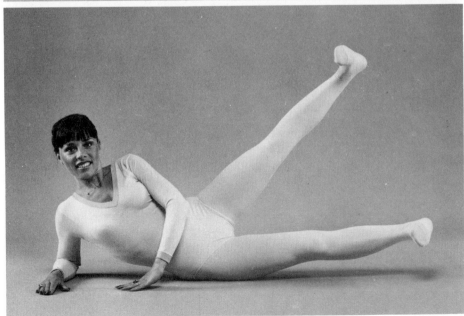

3

Flex your feet. Raise and lower your left leg 8 times, still keeping your right leg 6 inches off the floor. Change sides and repeat with the right leg.

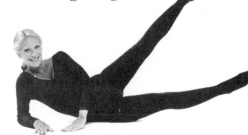

Stem Lift

For best results, keep your torso straight and your feet pointed. This is an excellent exercise for keeping your hips firm.

Suzy's Program

First through third month: complete sequence once

Fourth through six month: repeat sequence twice

Seventh through ninth month: repeat sequence once

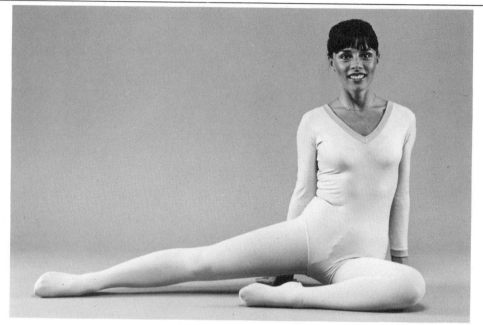

1

Sit with your left leg bent in front of you and your right leg stretched out to the side. Place your hands on the floor behind your fanny.

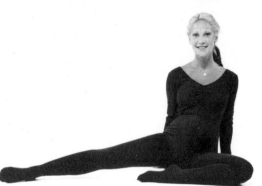

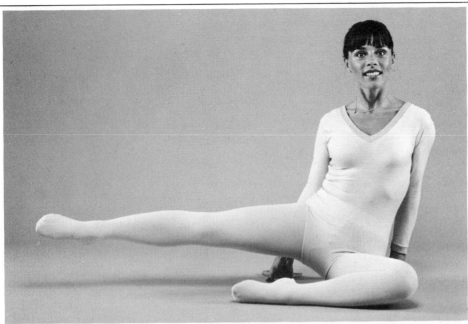

2

Without leaning too far to the left, raise and lower your right leg 8 times. Keep your leg straight and your knee facing forward.

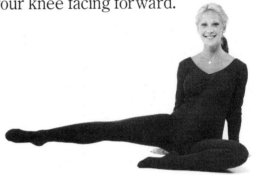

3

Change sides and repeat with your left leg.

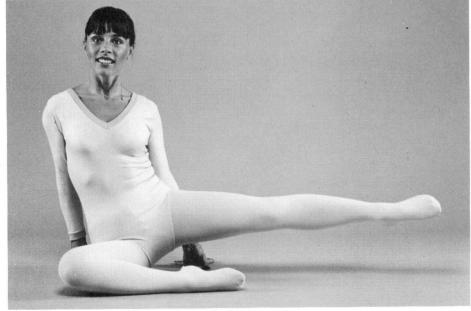

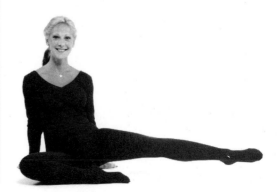

Cross-legged Breathing

This exercise not only relaxes your body and mind, but the cross-legged position helps to stretch your inner thigh muscles. Additionally, breath control will add to the control of muscles during delivery.

Suzy's Program

First through ninth month: repeat sequence at least 6 times, once a day, and whenever you feel tense and wish to relax

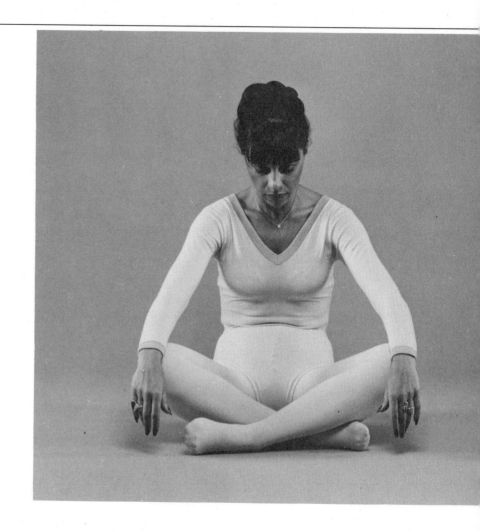

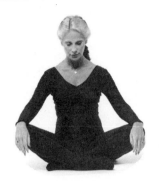

1

Sit on the floor with your legs bent and crossed in front of you. Place the undersides of your forearms and wrists on your knees, and relax your hands.

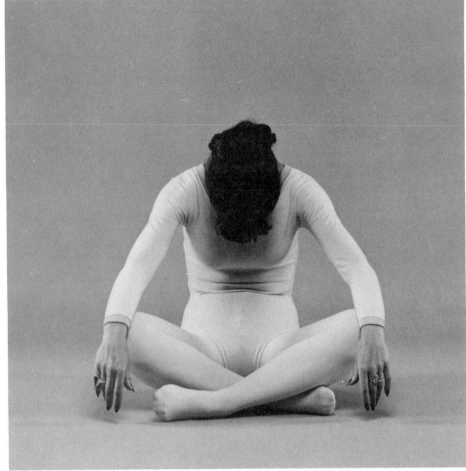

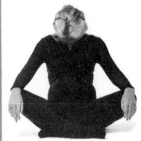

2

Close your eyes and round your back slightly, letting your head gently drop forward. Inhale through your nose to the count of 4, then exhale to the count of 4.

77

Straight-leg Breathing

In order to protect your lower back, it is important to keep one leg bent, while raising and lowering your straight leg.

Suzy's Program

First through third month: repeat sequence 6 times

Fourth through sixth month: repeat sequence 8 times

Seventh through ninth month: repeat sequence 6 times

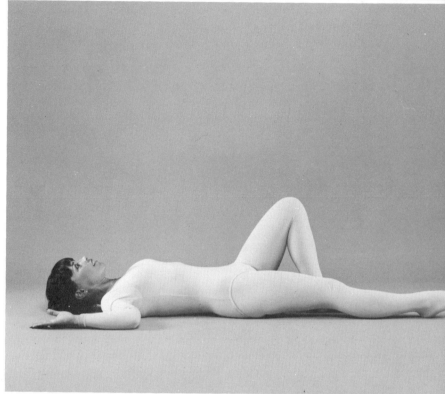

1

Lie on your back with your forearms parallel to your head. Bend your left leg at the knees, keeping the sole of your left foot flat on the floor. Your right leg is straight, with your foot pointed.

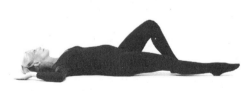

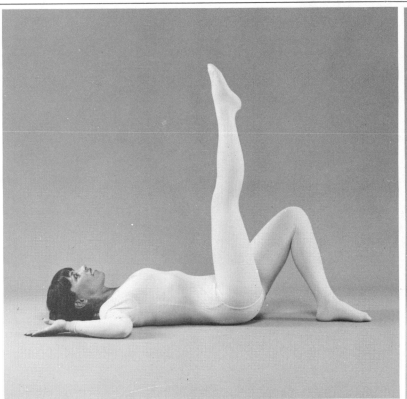

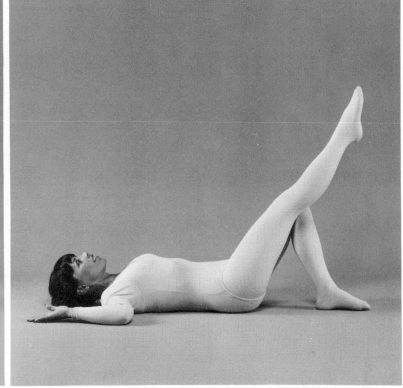

2

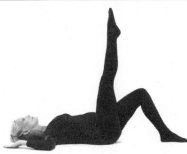

Without moving your left leg, lift your right leg so that it is perpendicular to the floor. As you do so, press your lower back against the floor and inhale to the count of 4.

3

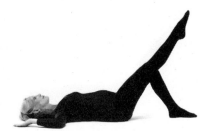

Slowly exhale to the count of 4, while you lower your right leg. Repeat with your other leg.

Chair Shrug

This is another exercise that can be done anywhere you are sitting. It is particularly effective for relaxing stiff necks and tense shoulders.

Suzy's Program

First through ninth month: repeat sequence at least 10 times, once a day, and whenever you want to relax your neck and shoulders

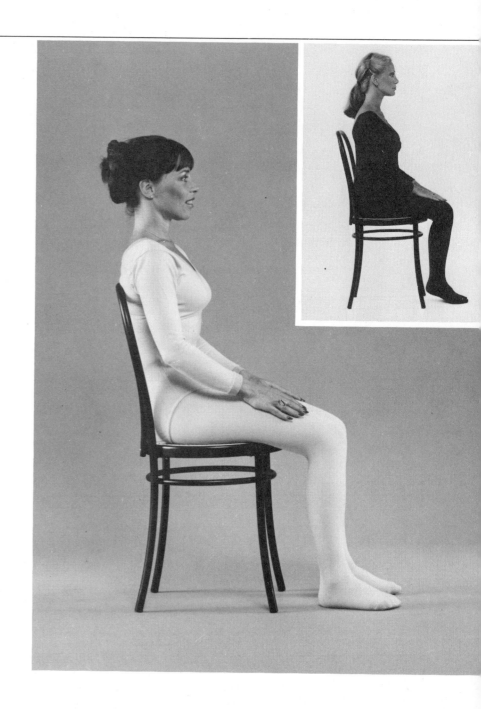

1

Sit on a straight-backed chair. Press your lower back against the back of the chair and tighten your stomach muscles.

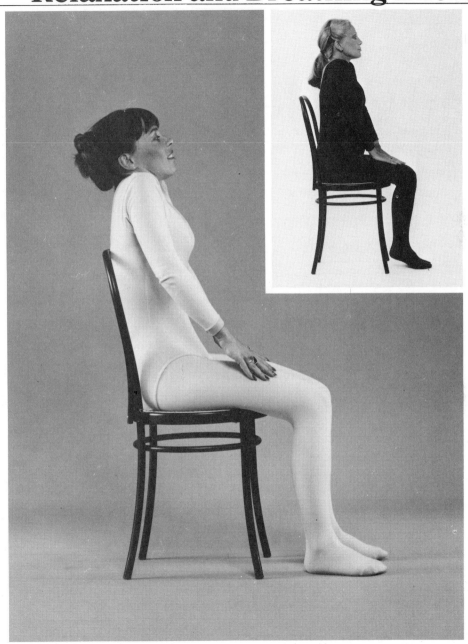

2

While inhaling to the count of 4, raise your shoulders toward your ears. Then exhale and lower your shoulders to the count of 4.

Head Circle

An old, but proven effective, exercise for relaxing your neck, shoulders, and upper back. However, if you experience any dizziness, stop and sit down.

Suzy's Program

First through ninth month: repeat sequence 6 times, and whenever your neck and upper back are stiff and tense

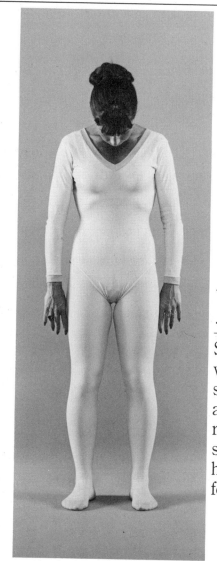

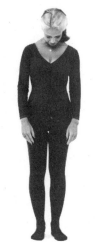

1

Stand straight with your legs slightly apart and your arms relaxed at your sides. Let your head drop forward.

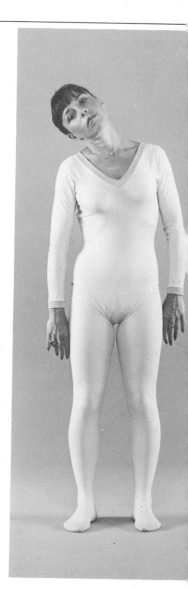

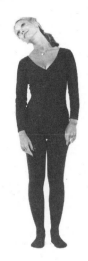

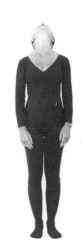

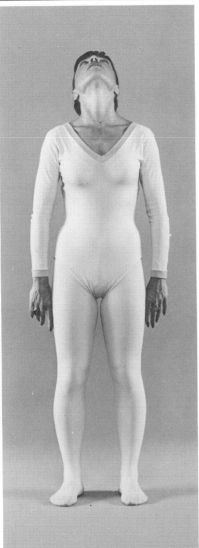

2

Rotate your head to the right, letting your chin pass over your right shoulder.

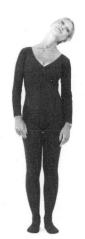

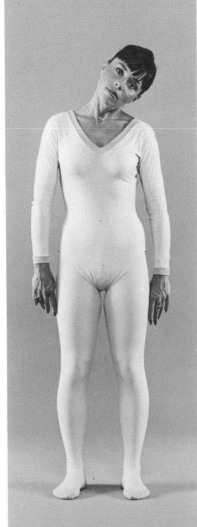

3

Continue to rotate your head to the back and look straight up at the ceiling.

4

Rotate your head over your left shoulder and return to your original position. Repeat rotation in the opposite direction.

Shoulder Circle

This simple exercise is utilized by athletes to add flexibility to their shoulders and arms. It is highly relaxing and good for relieving tension.

Suzy's Program

First through ninth month: repeat sequence 8 times, once a day, and whenever you experience tightness in your shoulders and upper back.

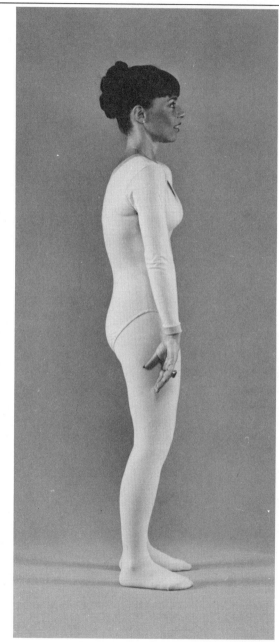

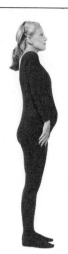

1

Stand with your legs slightly apart, your arms relaxed at your sides, and your stomach muscles tightened. Begin a rotating motion by rounding your shoulders forward.

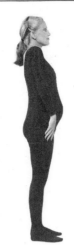

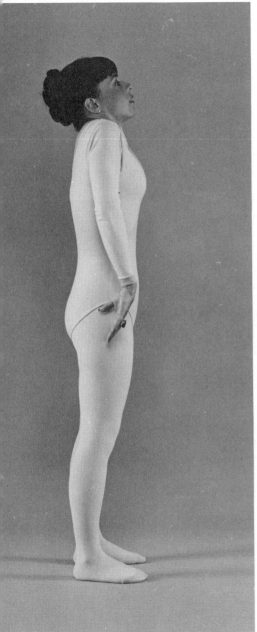

2

Lift your shoulders toward your ears, still keeping your stomach muscles tightened.

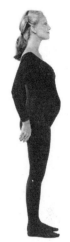

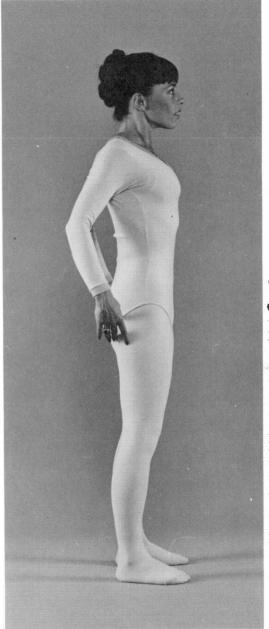

3

Stretch your shoulders back as far as possible. Relax your stomach muscles and lower your shoulders to their original position. Repeat rotation in the opposite direction.

Sitting "C"

In order for this exercise to be effective, you should not bend forward from the waist. Your upper shoulder should be thrust slightly backward to keep your torso straight.

Suzy's Program

First through third month: complete sequence once

Fourth through six month: repeat sequence twice

Seventh through ninth month: repeat sequence 3 times

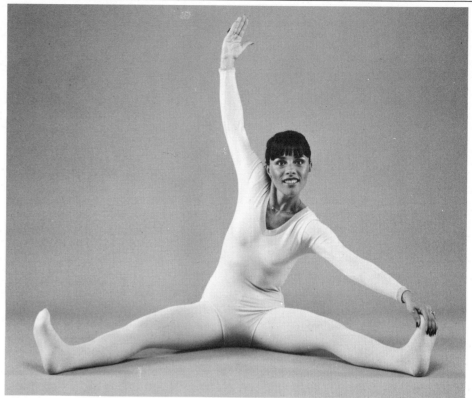

1

Sit with your legs straight and spread as far apart as possible, with your knees facing the ceiling and feet flexed. Hold your left foot with your left hand, and raise your right arm straight over your head.

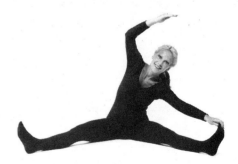

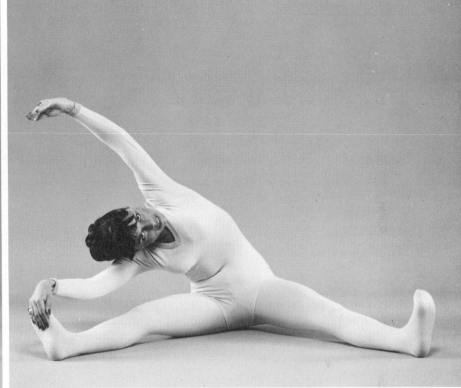

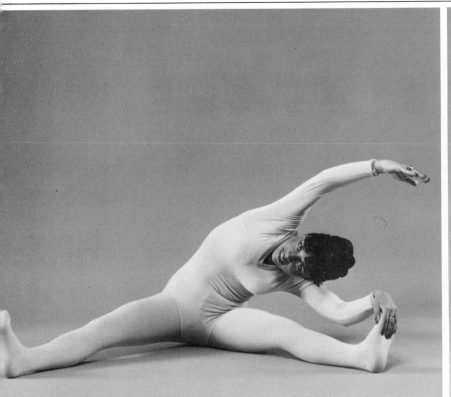

2

Stretch your right arm to the left, making an arc of your body. Bounce your torso and arm 8 times to the left. Do not lower your right shoulder and be sure to continue to face forward.

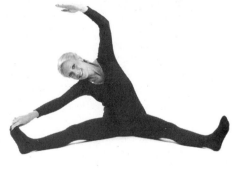

3

Reverse the position of your arms. Stretch your left arm and torso to the right without lowering your left shoulder. Bounce your torso and arm 8 times to the right.

Up Thrust

In addition to helping you stay flexible throughout your pregnancy, this exercise will also strengthen your thighs, arms, shoulders, and back. You may find the exercise too difficult to do after your sixth month; if so, do not do the exercise.

Suzy's Program

First through third month: repeat sequence 4 times

Fourth through sixth month: repeat sequence 6 times

Seventh through ninth month: repeat sequence 4 times unless you find it too difficult

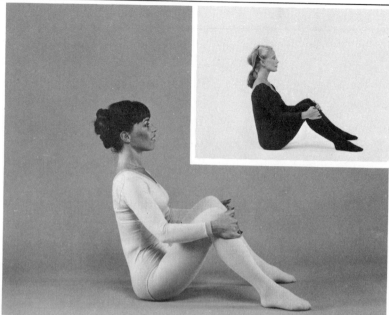

1

Sit with your knees bent and feet as far apart as is comfortable. Clasp your knees with your hands and keep your feet flat on the floor.

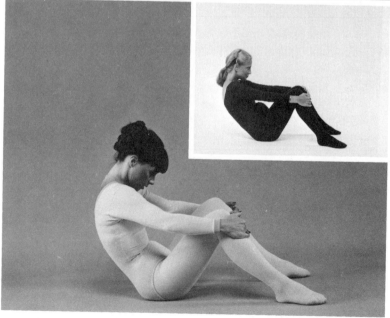

2

Tighten your stomach muscles, round your back, and tilt your head forward.

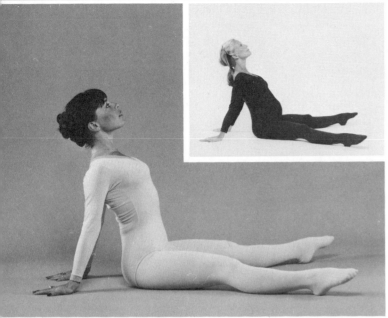

3

Place your hands on the floor behind your fanny and stretch your legs out in front of you, feet apart and pointed. Arch your back slightly.

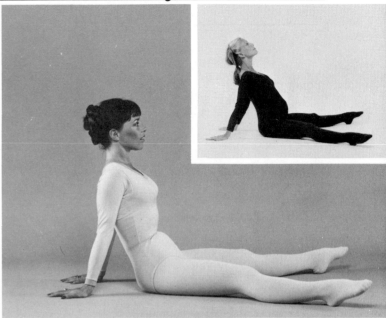

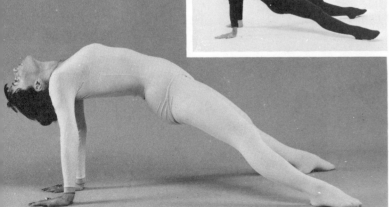

4

Lift your fanny off the floor and straighten your torso. Stretch your neck and allow your head to fall back. Hold this position for 4 seconds.

5

Lower your torso and fanny to a sitting position.

"L"-shaped Body

This exercise is particularly effective for stretching the muscles in the inner thighs and backs of legs; if not stretched, these areas may have a tendency to ache and cramp during pregnancy. Stretching the inner thighs will also help during delivery.

Suzy's Program

First through third month:
repeat sequence twice

Fourth through sixth month:
repeat sequence 4 times

Seventh through ninth month:
repeat sequence 6 times

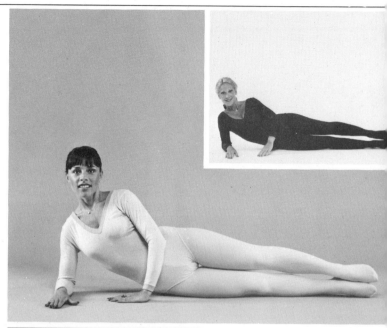

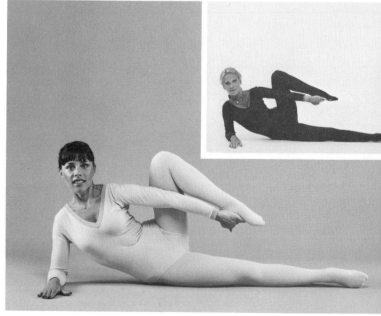

1

Lie on your right side with your torso propped up on your right elbow and your left hand resting in front. Your legs should be straight and feet pointed.

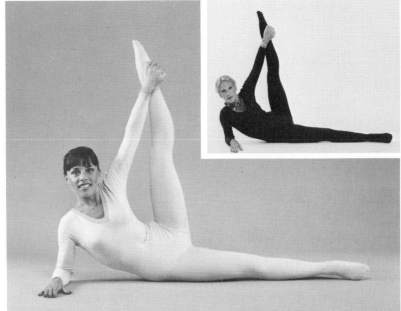

2

Bend your left leg. With your left hand, clasp the arch of your left foot. If you cannot reach the arch, then clasp your calf. Your elbow should be against the inner thigh, and your knee should face the ceiling.

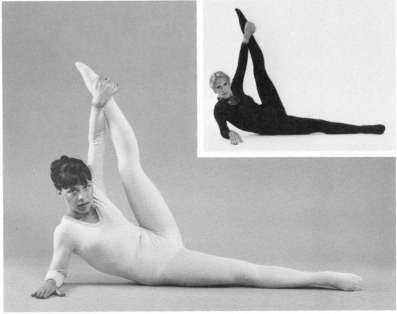

3

Still holding your left foot, straighten your left leg so it is perpendicular to the floor. Do not lean back, and hold this position for 4 seconds, then bend your knee.

4

Straighten and bend your left leg for a total of 4 times; on the fourth time you straighten your leg, pull it toward your left shoulder and, keeping it straight, bounce the leg 4 times toward the shoulder. Change sides and repeat with your right leg.

Rag Doll

When you finish this exercise, bring your head and torso up slowly so that you do not get dizzy. And when bent over, don't attempt to stretch farther than you comfortably can or you might put too much pressure on your stomach and strain your back and upper thighs.

Suzy's Program

First through ninth month: complete sequence at least once a day

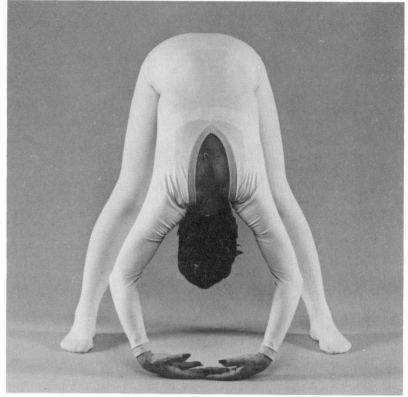

1

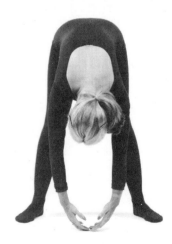

Stand with your legs straight, feet apart, and torso bent forward from the hips. Let your arms dangle in front of you so that your fingers can touch the floor. Bounce your torso toward the floor 8 times.

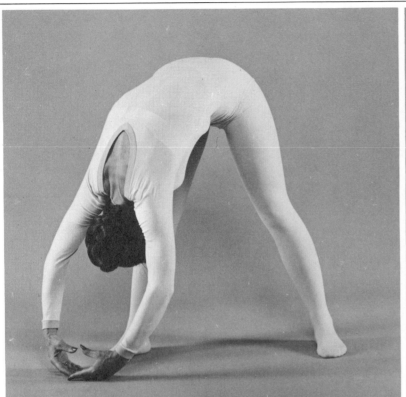

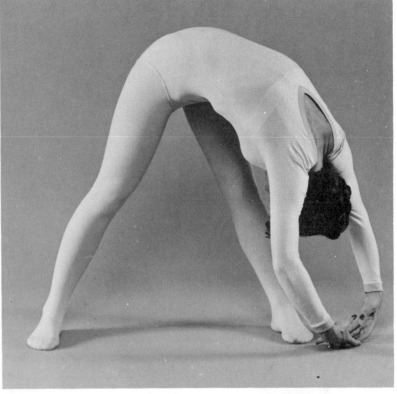

2

Turn your torso over your right leg and bounce 8 times.

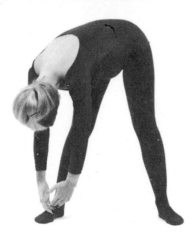

3

Turn your torso over your left leg and bounce 8 times, keeping both legs straight.

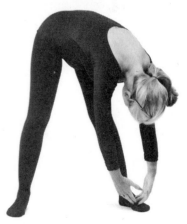

The Choreo-graphed Stretch

This exercise may seem long and complicated at first, but as you learn the order of the movements you'll be able to perform them smoothly. End your exercise session with this stretch, which will loosen your muscles and leave your entire body thoroughly relaxed.

Suzy's Program

First through ninth month:
repeat sequence 3 times

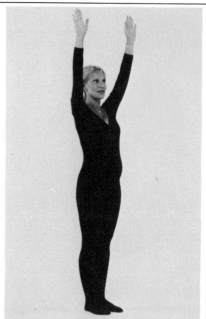

1

Stand with your legs straight, feet together, and arms stretched straight up above your head.

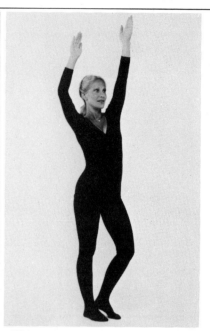

2

Bend your left knee slightly and stretch your left arm over your head. Straighten your left knee and relax your left arm, but don't lower it. Repeat with the right side. Stretch each arm 8 times, alternating.

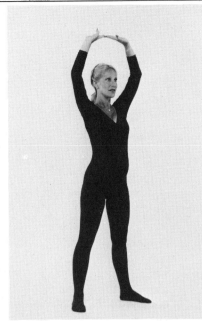
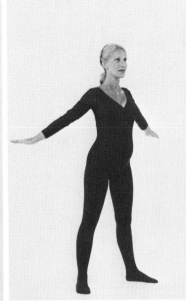
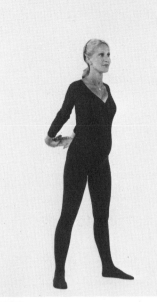
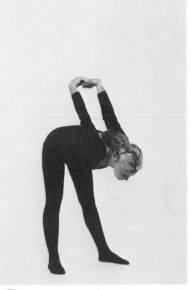

3

Spread your feet apart and arch your arms over your head so the tips of your fingers touch and your palms face upward. Do not arch your back.

4

Pull your hands apart, and lower your arms to a count of 4. Keep your hands pointing upward.

5

Clasp your hands tightly behind your fanny.

6

Bend your torso forward from the hips, raising your arms as high as you can above your back. Bounce forward 4 times.

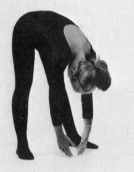 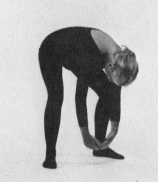 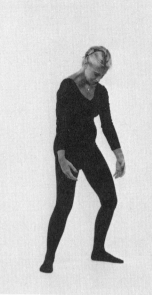 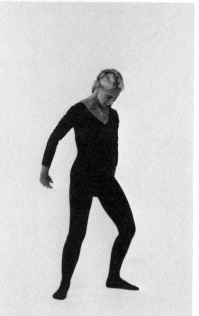

7

Unclasp your hands and let your arms dangle in front of your legs. Bounce forward with straight legs 4 times.

8

Bend your knees and tuck your pelvis forward.

9

Slowly straighten your torso, keeping your knees bent.

10

As your body straightens, your hands should fall behind your fanny.

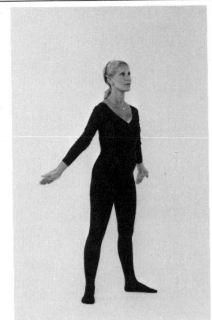

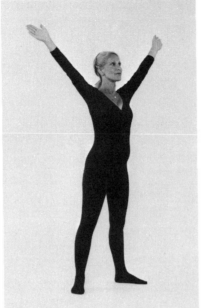

11

Straighten your
legs, stretch
your arms
behind you, and
arch your upper
back.

12

Raise your
straight arms
over your head
and bring your
feet together.
This will bring
you to the
original starting
position.

Sitting, Chin Forward

This is a superb exercise for stretching the muscles in your calves and thighs. However, as your stomach grows larger, be careful not to press it against your leg. Stretch slowly and cautiously.

Suzy's Program

First through third month: repeat sequence 6 times

Fourth through six month: repeat sequence 8 times

Seventh through ninth month: repeat sequence 10 times

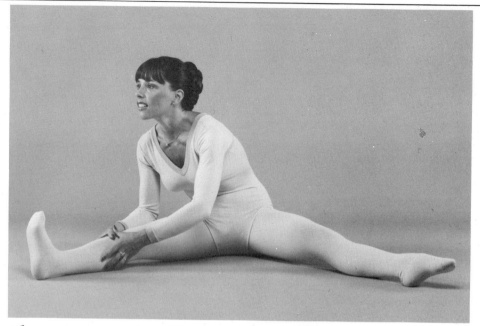

1

Sit with your legs wide apart and stretched out straight. With both hands, clasp your right leg below the knee and flex your right foot. Your left foot should be pointed and both knees facing the ceiling.

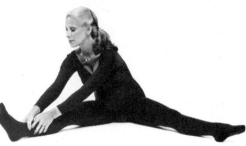

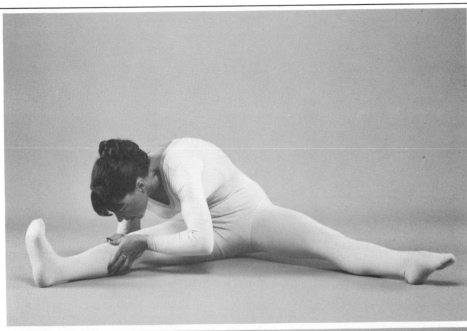

2

Without bending your knees, slowly pull your torso over your right leg and try to touch your chin to your right knee. Do not strain. Hold this position for 8 seconds.

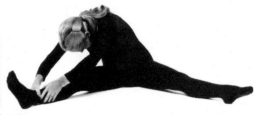

3

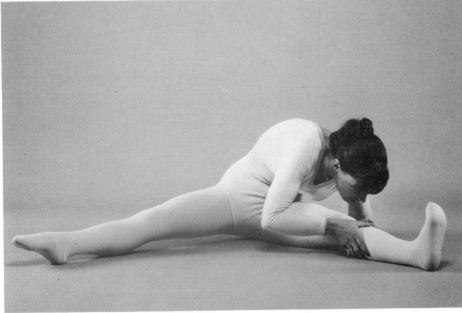

In the same manner, pull your torso over your left leg and hold for 8 seconds.

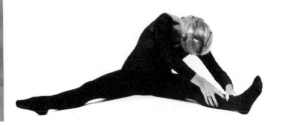

99

Wall Stretch

This is a particularly important exercise to help prepare you for delivery because it stretches the inner thigh muscles. The more you do it, the easier it will become. You may wish to place a small pillow beneath your head and read an absorbing book.

Suzy's Program

First through ninth month: complete exercise at least once a day

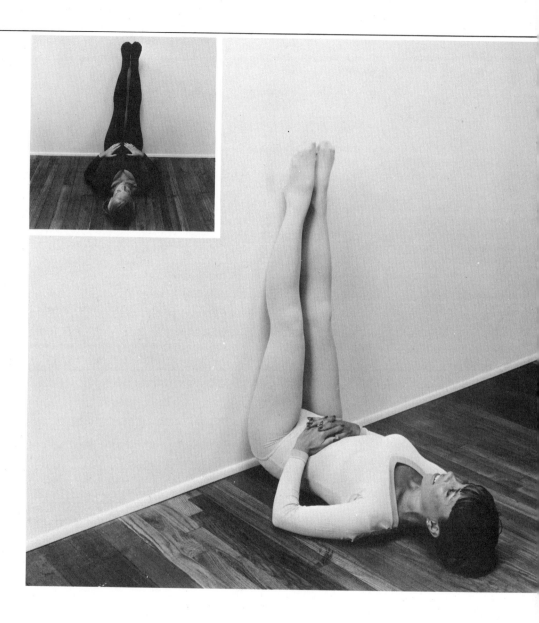

1

Lie on the floor so that the bottom of your fanny is pressed against a wall. Your legs should be straight and placed against the wall to form a right angle with your body.

2

Slowly spread your legs as far apart as you can. Keep your back flat on the floor and remain in this position for 5 to 10 minutes.

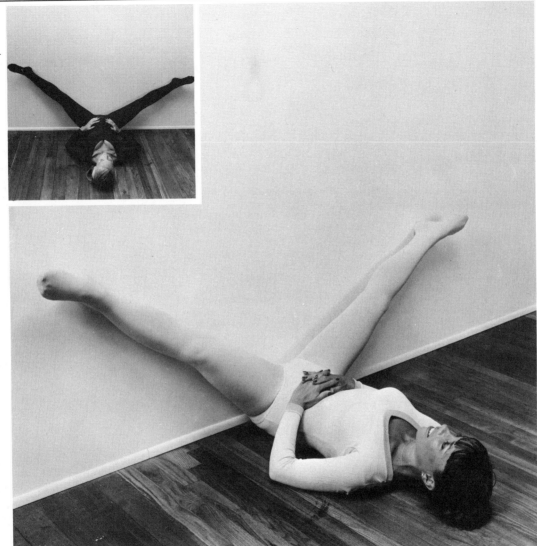

Against the Wall

Another very effective exercise for stretching the inner thigh muscles and for preparing muscles for delivery.

Suzy's Program

First through third month: repeat sequence 4 times

Fourth through sixth month: repeat sequence 8 times

Seventh through ninth month: repeat sequence 12 times

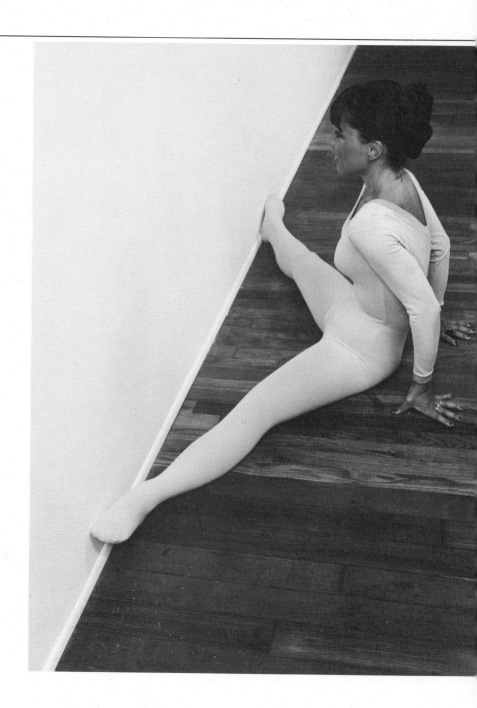

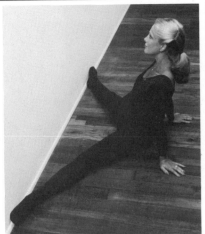

1

Sit on the floor
and spread your
legs as far apart
as possible with
feet pointed and
touching the
wall. Your legs
should be
straight, knees
facing the
ceiling. Place
your palms on
the floor directly
behind your
fanny.

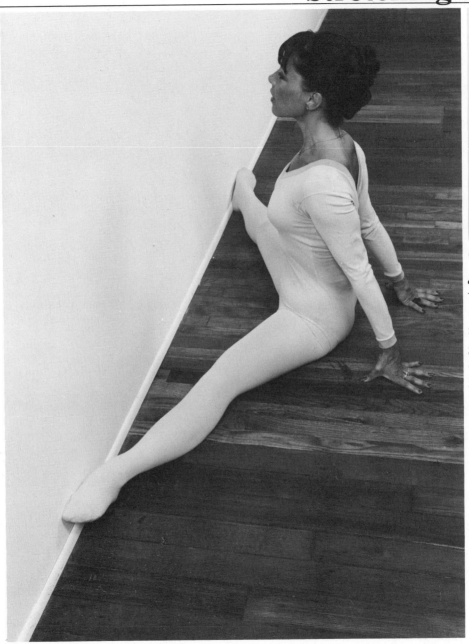

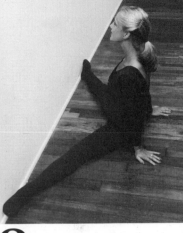

2

Hold your torso
straight and
attempt to push
your pelvis
toward the wall.
Hold 60 seconds,
then relax.

Bridging the Gap

Although this exercise seems difficult, it is quite easy if you balance yourself on your hands. It is excellent for stretching the pelvic region.

Suzy's Program

First through third month: repeat sequence 4 times

Fourth through sixth month: repeat sequence 8 times

Seventh through ninth month: repeat sequence 12 times

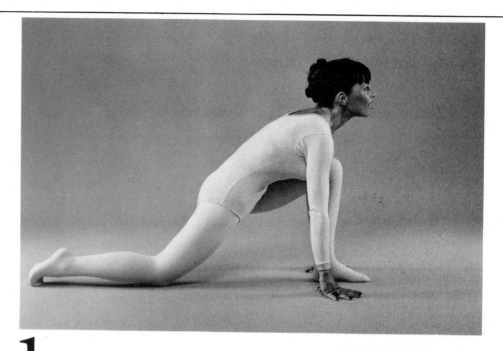

1

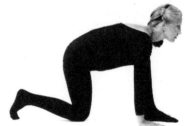

Beginning on your hands and knees, place your left foot next to the inside of your left hand.

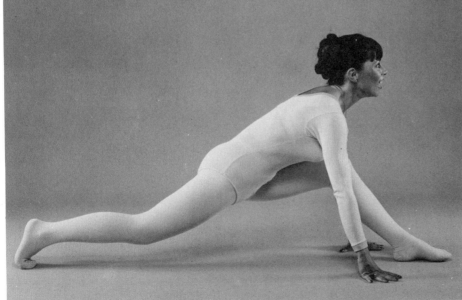

2

Keeping your left leg in place, stretch your right leg out behind you as far as possible, so that it rests on the ball of the foot.

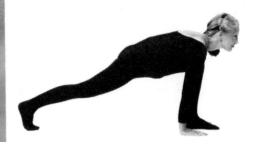

3

Move your left leg forward several inches, keeping your foot flat on the floor. Your right leg should bend slightly at the knee. Hold for 4 seconds. Change legs and repeat.

Bent-leg Stretch

This exercise stretches the muscles in the backs of the thighs. It should be done slowly to prevent unnecessary strain. Spread your legs as wide as you comfortably can.

Suzy's Program

Second through third month: repeat sequence twice

Fourth through sixth month: repeat sequence 4 times

Seventh through ninth month: repeat sequence 8 times

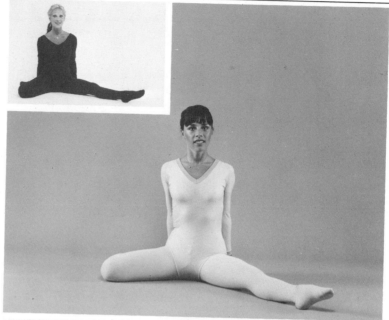

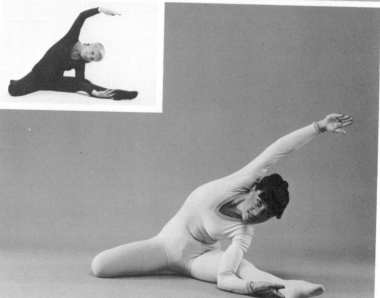

1

Sit with your left leg stretched straight out to the left, foot pointed. Your right leg should be bent so that your right foot points backward and rests on the floor in back of your fanny. Place your hands on the floor behind your fanny and push your pelvis forward.

2

Raise your right arm and place your left hand under your left calf. Stretch your torso toward your left leg. Hold for 8 seconds.

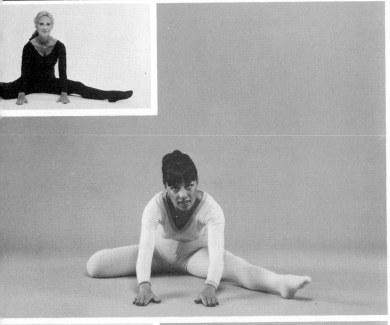

3

Release your left leg, lower your right arm, and stretch out both arms, palms down, in front of you.

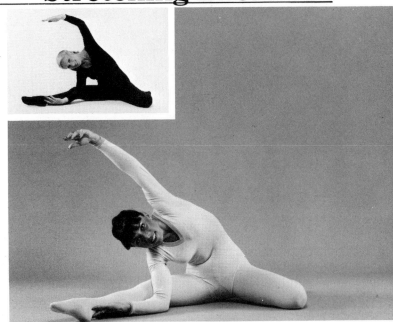

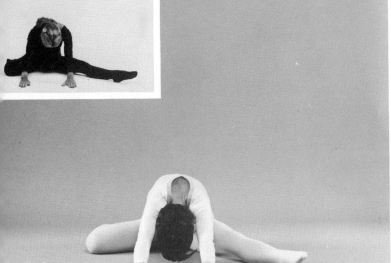

4

Stretch your arms straight out as far as possible, bending your torso toward the floor. Hold this position for 12 seconds.

5

Repeat with your right leg stretched out.

Phone Book Stretch

A simple but particularly effective exercise for stretching the backs of the calves and the Achilles tendon. It will make walking, especially up and down stairs, easier than it otherwise might be.

Suzy's Program

First through ninth month: repeat sequence 12 times, and whenever you experience tightness in the backs of your calves

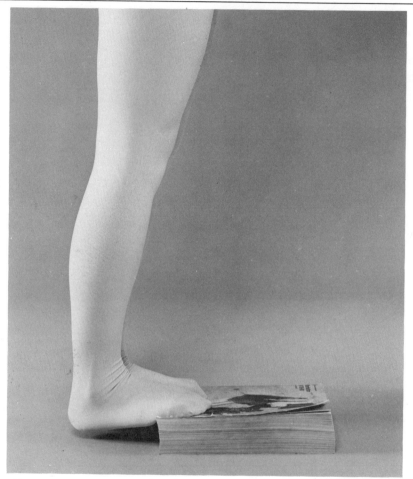

1

Hold on to a chair or couch for balance and place your toes and the balls of your feet on a thick book, such as a phone directory.

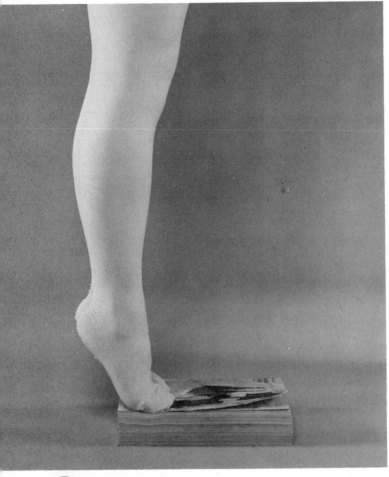

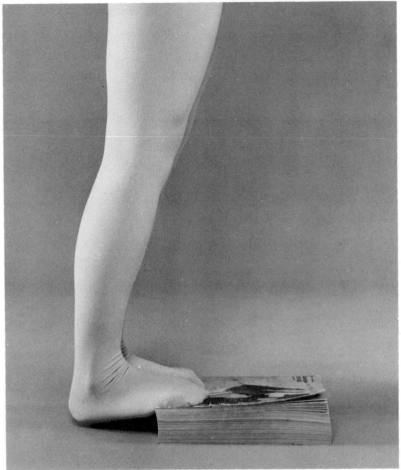

2

Lift up on your toes and hold for 2 seconds.

3

Lower your feet and press your heels toward the floor and hold for 16 seconds.

Postpartum Program

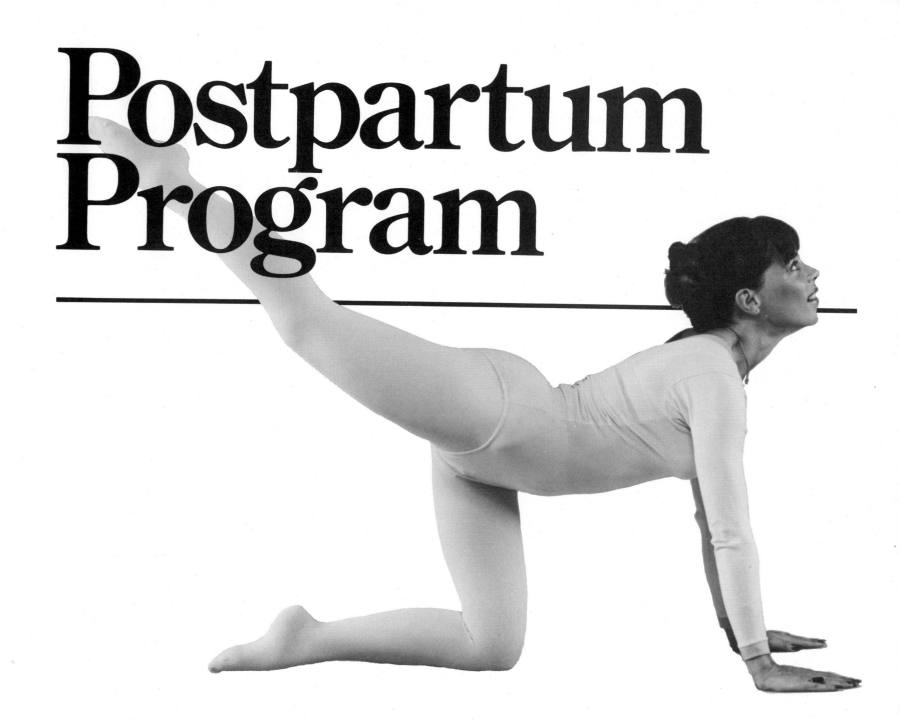

Before beginning the pregnancy exercises, you had a complete physical examination and were given your doctor's permission to undertake our program of pregnancy exercises. You should do the same before embarking on the exercises in the postpartum section of this book.

Some women are ready to start exercising a few days after they have returned home from the hospital; others want to do nothing but lie in bed and relax for a couple of weeks. If you experienced complications during your delivery, you may require even more time for rest and recuperation. In any case, you should start your exercise program slowly and gently, aiming at restoring yourself to an optimum level of fitness and health.

After resting from labor and delivery, women are primed to get their bodies back into shape. Just as the internal organs are already restoring themselves to their pre-pregnant condition, the voluntary muscles are waiting for you to tone, tighten, and strengthen them.

The muscles most obviously in need of conditioning are the abdominals—and no wonder: they have been stretched out of shape for nine months! However, they will not require nine months of exercise to become flattened and toned again. The body is marvelously responsive, ready to go in any direction you send it, and the stomach exercises in this section will help you to have the flat stomach you want.

Though you cannot see the muscles of the pelvic floor, they have also been severely stretched during delivery. A sign of this may be that you suffer from loss of sphincter control during elimination. Don't worry, this can be corrected. In addition, the vaginal muscles have been stretched, and they require isometric exercises so you can enjoy sexual intercourse again. You should do the pelvic exercises in the pregnancy section as part of your postpartum program for both these problems.

During the lactation period, your breasts will grow quite large and heavy. Without strong pectoral muscles and the proper kind of bra, they may also become unnecessarily pendulous, and can leave you with unattractive stretch marks. You should do all the pectoral exercises in this section, as well as those in the pregnancy section. Remember to wear a bra, especially when exercising or engaging in sports.

Once you are up and around, you may find that your feet hurt and that you experience spasms or cramps in your upper and lower legs. These problems are probably caused by lack of exercise and poor circulation. The leg exercises here will not only keep your legs strong and shapely, but they will enhance circulation and mitigate the problems of foot pains and cramped muscles. Furthermore, if you exercise your legs regularly, you will be able to diminish the size and number of varicose veins. That does not mean that exercise alone will eliminate them; it only means that varicosity may be decreased by improved circulation.

During pregnancy, your posture had to make a number of adjustments to accommodate your growing stomach. Now that you are no longer front-heavy, you will have to make other adjustments so that you stand straight and do not experience lower back pain. Be very conscious of the way you hold and carry yourself. Be straight, but be comfortable; there is no virtue in standing rigidly. You will find that the exercises for the back will be of inestimable value in helping restore your posture.

Many women suffer from what is commonly called postpartum blues. There are many reasons for these feelings of depression, but once those blues have become a little pink around the edges, there is nothing better than a regular fitness program for wiping them away altogether.

The exercises in this section serve a variety of purposes. Some of the exercises are strictly for spot reducing, to tone and trim areas that increased in bulk and weight during pregnancy. Others will instill energy, warding off fatigue, irritability, and the blues. And others will contribute to your overall recuperation often accelerating what would otherwise take a long time.

Positive results will begin to be apparent after several weeks, and your goals may be achieved within a few months. Those results include a refreshed level of energy, restored self-esteem, and a body that is healthy, strong, and fit.

General rules you should follow:

- Have a complete medical examination and do only those exercises that your doctor says you can do right away.
- Begin slowly and gently, for you will not know how much you can do when you first start.
- Never exert yourself to the point of exhaustion, pain, or dizziness. When your body feels tired, stop. You have had enough.
- Exercise regularly. Consistency will reward you with the results you desire.
- If you ever feel nausea, dizzy, or ill, stop exercising and consult your doctor.
- Breathe regularly while exercising. Never hold your breath. Do not exhale, then forget to inhale.
- Read each step of the exercises and do them carefully.
- Do all recumbent exercises on a cushiony towel, blanket, or mat.

Classic Sit-up

If you have any difficulty raising your torso off the floor with your hands clasped behind your neck, stretch your arms over your head and swing them up along with your torso. After a few weeks, try the exercise with your hands clasped behind your neck.

Suzy's Program

Third through seventh week: repeat sequence 4 times

Eighth through twelfth week: repeat sequence 8 times

Thereafter: repeat sequence 12 times

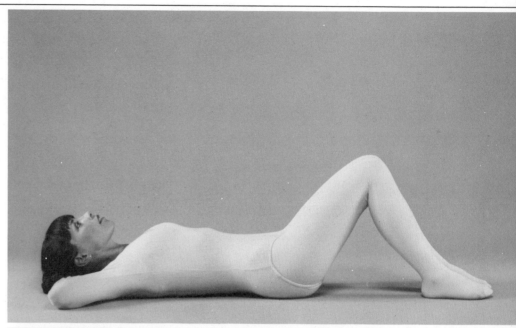

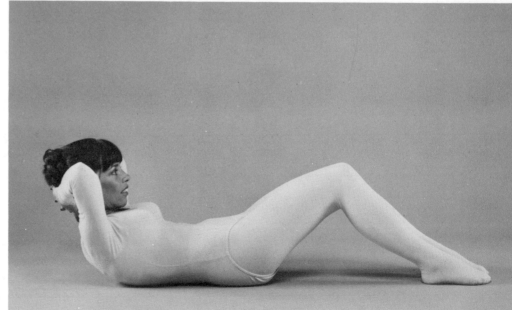

1

Lie flat on your back with knees bent and feet flat on the floor. Clasp your hands behind your neck or stretch them out on the floor behind your neck.

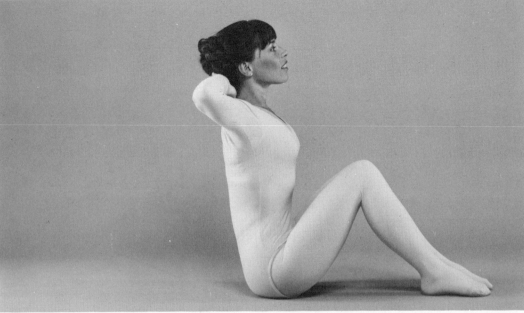

2

Tighten your stomach muscles and slowly bring your torso up into a sitting position, with your back rounded. Keep your feet flat on the floor.

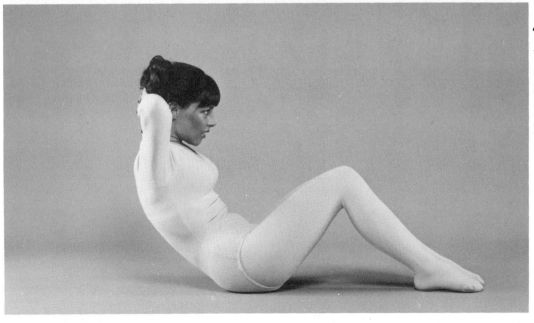

3

When you reach a sitting position, straighten your back, keeping your stomach pulled in and your knees pressed together. Hold this position for 4 seconds.

4

Round your back and slowly lower your torso to the floor.

Round Back and Straighten

This exercise is similar to the one you did during your pregnancy, but here it is done with your legs and feet together.

Suzy's Program

Third through seventh week: repeat sequence 8 times

Eighth through twelfth week: repeat sequence 12 times

Thereafter: repeat sequence 16 times

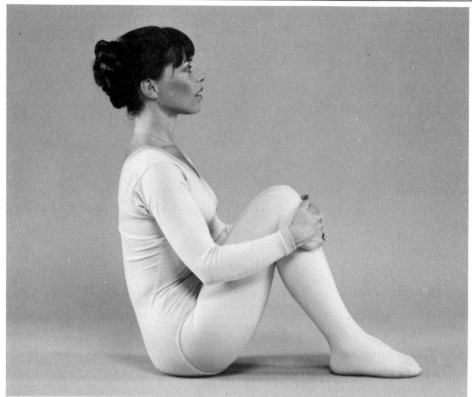

1

Sit with your knees bent and your feet flat on the floor. Keep your legs together and clasp them with your hands below your knees.

116

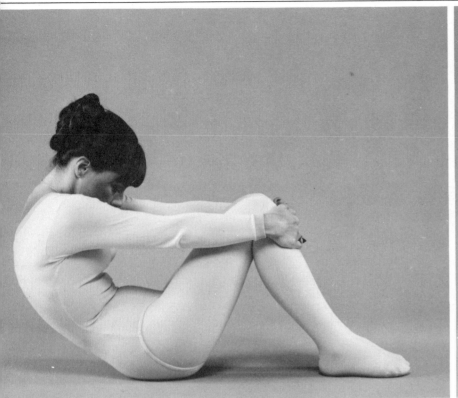

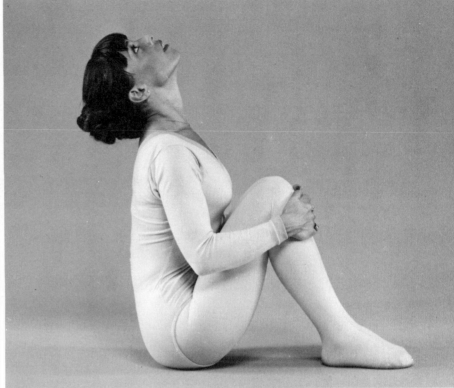

2

Round your back and let your head drop toward your chest. Your arms are extended and straight. Tighten your stomach muscles and hold this position for 4 seconds.

3

Slowly straighten your back, pushing your chest toward your knees. Lift your face toward the ceiling, stretching out the front of your neck. Keep your stomach muscles tightened. Hold for 4 seconds, then relax.

Supine Hip Lift

For best results, keep your back rounded as you lower your fanny, vertebra by vertebra. This exercise is excellent for strengthening your lower back as well as your stomach muscles.

Suzy's Program

Third through seventh week: repeat sequence 4 times

Eighth through twelfth week: repeat sequence 8 times

Thereafter: repeat sequence 12 times

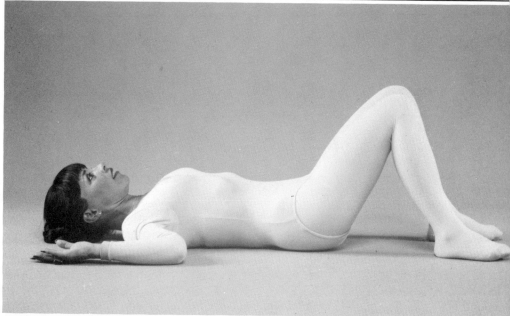

1

Lie on your back with knees bent. Your feet should be flat on the floor and about 8 inches apart. Bend your arms at the elbows so that your forearms are parallel to your head. Tighten your stomach muscles.

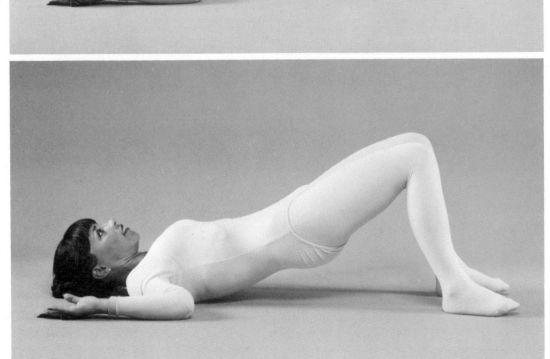

2

While raising your fanny off the floor, tuck your pelvis under. Hold this position for 4 seconds.

3

Keeping your pelvis tucked under, slowly lower your body, vertebra by vertebra, to the floor.

On-elbows Scissors

In addition to strengthening your stomach and lower back muscles, this exercise also helps trim your inner and outer thighs. But if you experience any pain in your lower back, do not continue this exercise. Try it again after a few weeks of doing back exercises.

Suzy's Program

Third through seventh week: repeat sequence 3 times

Eighth through twelfth week: repeat sequence 8 times

Thereafter: repeat sequence 10 times

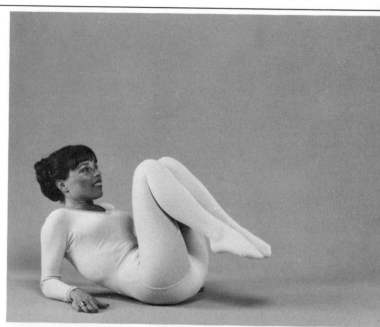

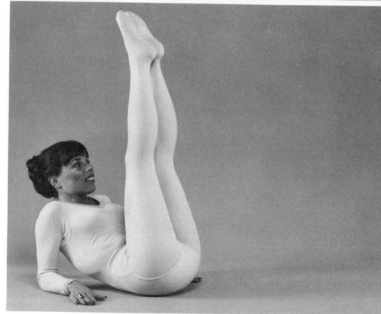

1

Sit on the floor and lean back on your elbows and forearms. Bend your knees over your chest and keep your feet pointed.

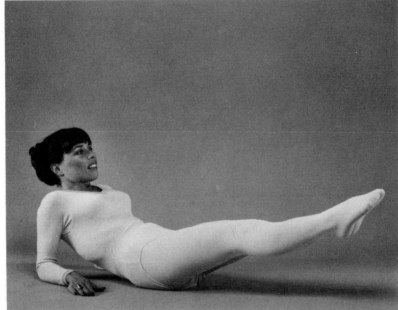

3

Tighten your stomach muscles and slowly lower your legs until they are about 10 inches off the floor. Keep your legs straight and your feet pointed.

2

Straighten your legs so that they are perpendicular to the floor.

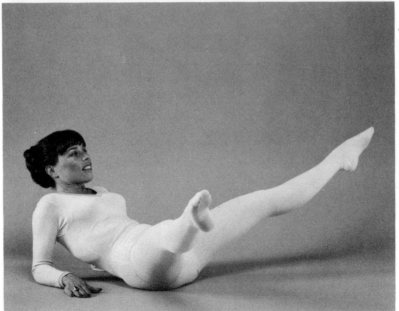

4

Open and close your legs 6 times, keeping your stomach muscles tightened. Then lower your legs to the floor.

On-elbows Bicycle

This effective exercise for strengthening stomach muscles is done during pregnancy and postpartum. Keep your legs pedaling in a continuous smooth motion and your stomach muscles tightened. After completing 8 pedaling motions with each leg, lean onto the right side of your fanny and pedal 8 more times with each leg. Then lean onto the left side, and pedal 8 times more with each leg.

Suzy's Program

Third through seventh week: complete sequence once

Thereafter: repeat sequence twice

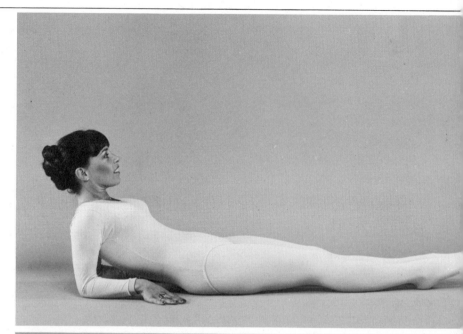

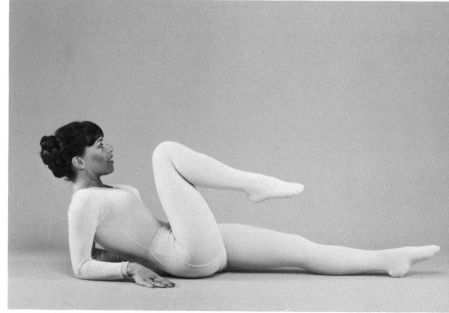

1

Lie on the floor with your torso propped up on your elbows. Your legs should be straight, feet together and pointed. Your forearms should be parallel to your body. Keep your hands flat on the floor.

2

Begin to bicycle by bending your right knee and bringing it up to your chest. Then, as you straighten the knee and lower your right leg, bend your left knee and bring it up to your chest.

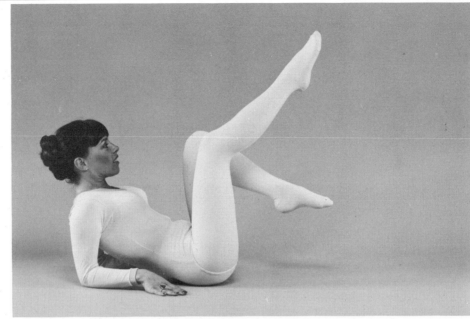

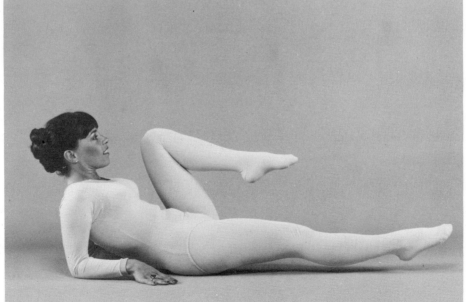

3

Continue this alternating movement, which should be like pedaling a bicycle. Keep your stomach muscles tightened.

4

Make 8 pedaling motions with each leg. Then lean onto first one side of your fanny and then the other, making 8 more pedaling motions on each side.

123

The Body Folds

This is one of the most effective exercises for flattening your stomach. You should make sure your back comes off the floor as your hands and feet stretch to meet. You may have to begin by doing only one sequence, but as your stomach muscles become stronger, you can work up to 10 sequences once a day.

Suzy's Program

Third through seventh week: repeat sequence twice

Eighth through twelfth week: repeat sequence 6 times

Thereafter: repeat sequence 10 times

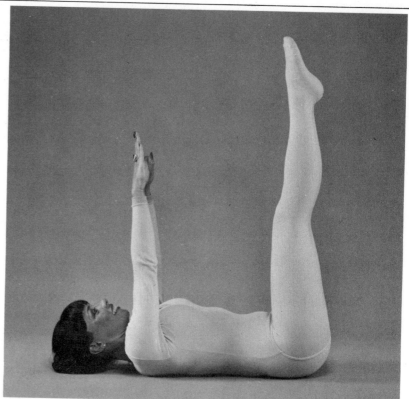

1

Lie flat on your back with your arms and legs stretched straight up in the air so that your body forms a "U." Your feet should be pointed.

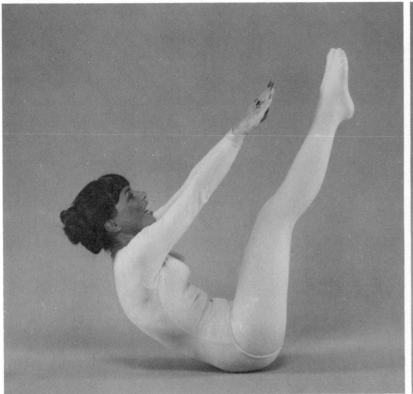

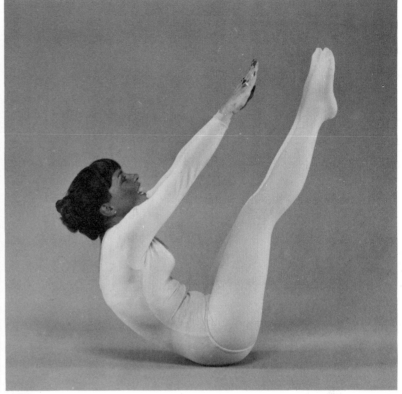

2

Keeping your stomach
pulled in, lift your back and
torso off the floor and
reach for your feet, all in
one movement.

3

Relax to the original
position, being sure to
keep your arms and legs
perpendicular to the floor.

Bent-leg Stem Lift

It is important to keep your body straight and lift your leg as high as you can.

Suzy's Program

Third through seventh week: repeat sequence 4 times

Eighth through twelfth week: repeat sequence 8 times

Thereafter: repeat sequence 12 times

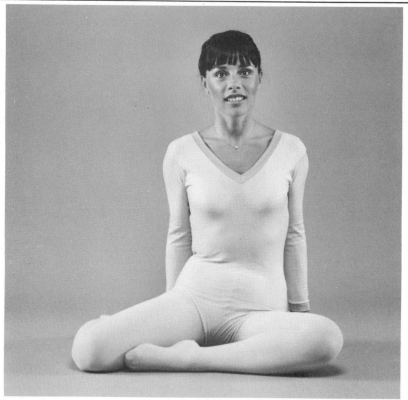

1

Sit with your left leg bent in front of you and your right leg bent so that your right foot points backward and rests on the floor in back of your fanny. Place your hands on the floor behind your fanny.

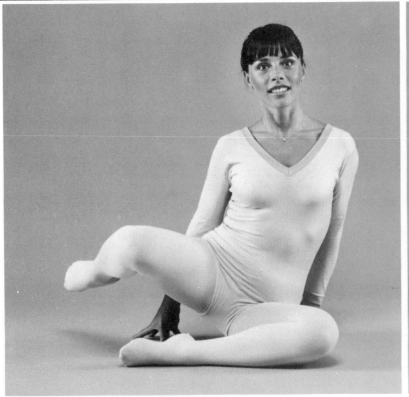

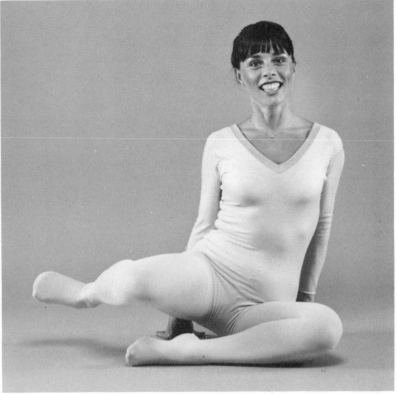

2

Raise and lower your right
leg 4 times with your foot
pointed.

3

Raise and lower your right
leg 4 times with your foot
flexed. Then repeat with
your left leg.

"Y" Kick-up

For best results, do this exercise lying on a hard surface. Lift your leg as high as you can, while trying to keep your hips parallel. If you feel strain in your lower back, raise your legs only 1 or 2 inches off the floor until your lower back muscles become strengthened.

Suzy's Program

Third through seventh week: repeat sequence twice

Eighth through twelfth week: repeat sequence 4 times

Thereafter: repeat sequence 7 times

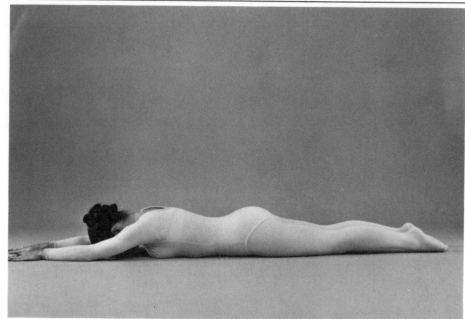

1

Lie on your stomach with your forehead resting on the floor and your arms stretched out in front. Tighten your stomach and fanny muscles.

2

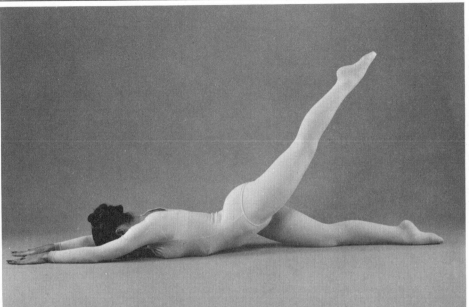

Lift your left leg as high off the floor as you can, keeping it straight with your foot pointed. Hold your leg in the air for 2 seconds, then slowly lower it to the floor.

3

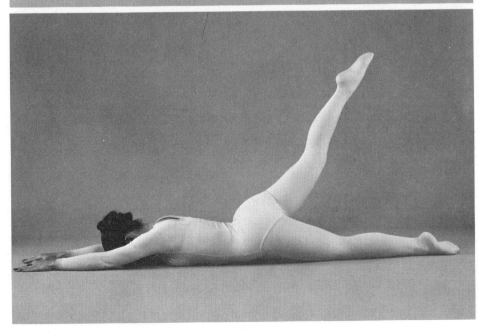

In the same manner, raise and lower your right leg.

Supine Air Kick

It is important to keep your lower back flat on the floor during this exercise—don't let it arch.

Suzy's Program

Third through seventh week: repeat sequence 8 times with each leg

Eighth through twelfth week: repeat sequence 12 times with each leg

Thereafter: repeat sequence 16 times with each leg

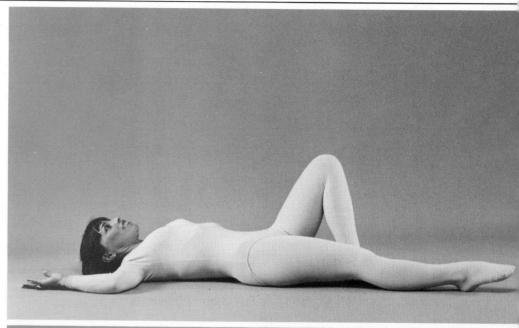

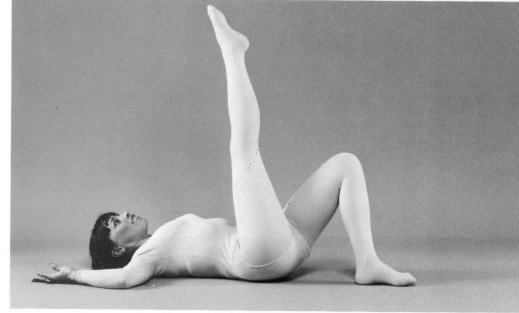

1

Lie on your back with your elbows bent and your forearms parallel to your head. Bend your left leg at the knee, keeping the sole of your left foot flat on the floor. Your right foot is pointed.

2

Without moving your left leg, raise your right leg until it is perpendicular to the floor. Keep your leg straight and your foot pointed.

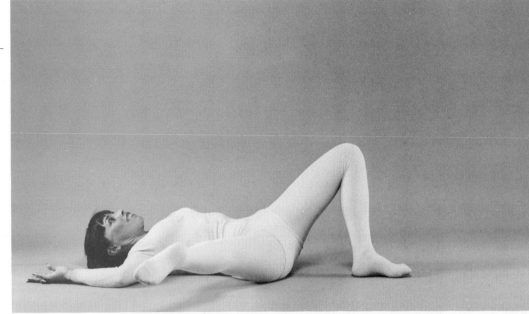

3

Lower your right leg out to the side until it is about 10 inches off the floor. Keep your left knee facing the ceiling.

4

Lift your leg up from the side until it is perpendicular to the floor.

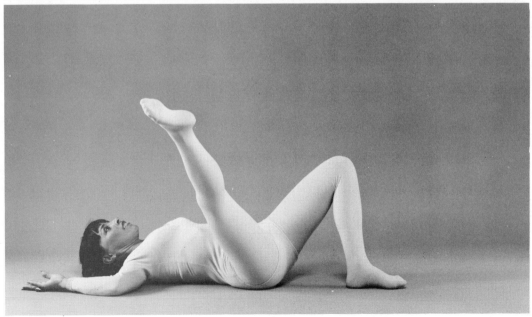

Baton Leg

Tightening your stomach and fanny muscles will help you keep your balance while you swing your leg backward and forward. Be sure to stretch your legs during this exercise.

Suzy's Program

Third through seventh week: complete sequence once

Eighth through twelfth week: repeat sequence twice

Thereafter: repeat sequence 3 times

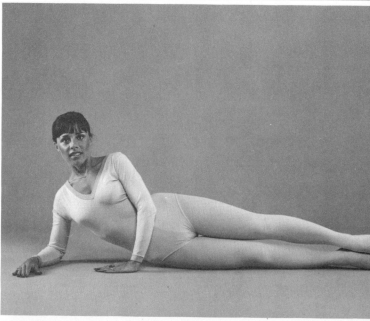

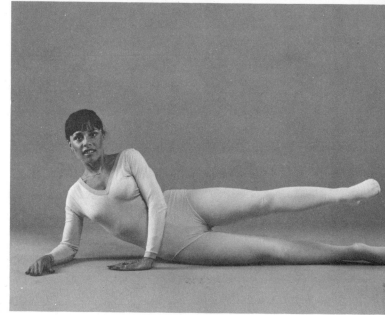

1

Lie on your right side with your torso propped up on your elbow and your left hand resting in front. Your legs should be straight and your feet pointed.

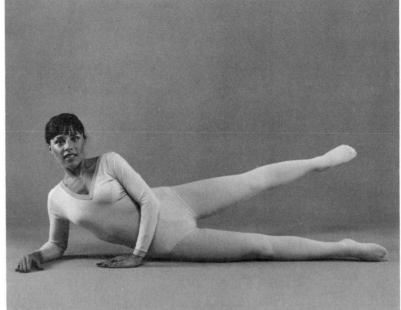

3

Swing your left leg forward, then backward, 4 times, keeping it straight and your torso still.

2

Lift your left leg about 6 inches off your right leg. Be sure knees face forward.

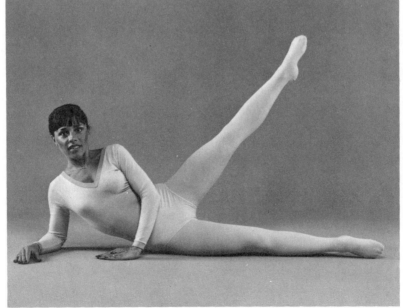

4

With your left leg, make 2 circles by moving it in a clockwise direction. Change sides and repeat with your left leg.

Orange Juice Squeeze

At first you may find it difficult to lift your leg more than a few inches off the floor. After a few weeks, however, your legs will be stronger and the exercise easier.

Suzy's Program

Third through seventh week: complete sequence once, with each leg

Eighth through twelfth week: repeat sequence 3 times, with each leg

Thereafter: repeat sequence 6 times, with each leg

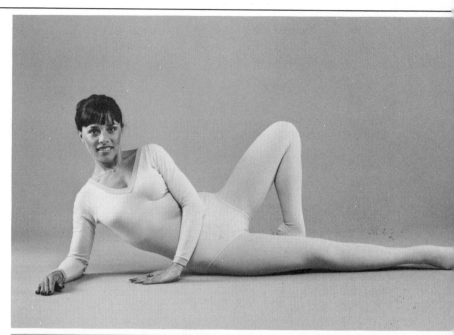

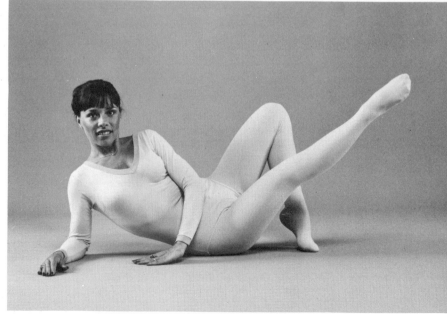

1

Lie on your right side with your torso propped up on your right elbow and your left hand resting in front. Bend your left leg so the ball of your left foot is on the floor behind your right knee. Keep your right leg straight, with foot pointed.

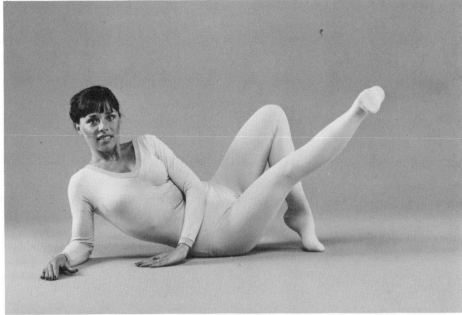

3

Flex your right foot.

2

Keeping your left hip off the floor, raise and lower your right leg 4 times with the foot pointed and knee facing forward. Lift your leg as high as you can, without leaning back on your fanny.

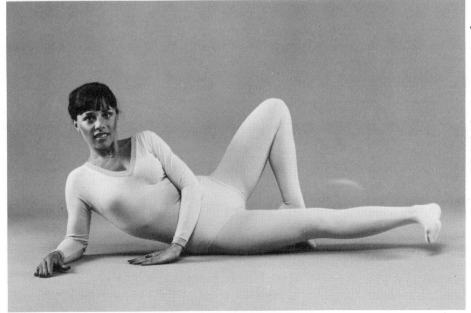

4

Raise and lower your right leg 4 times with your foot flexed and knee facing foward.

Cat Legs

Though this exercise looks easy, it is actually difficult—but excellent for the hips. Keep your toes pointed. Relax and stretch after completing the exercise.

Suzy's Program

Third through seventh week: repeat sequence twice with each leg

Eighth through twelfth week: repeat sequence 3 times with each leg

Thereafter: repeat sequence 4 times with each leg

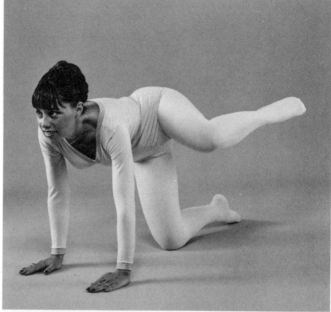

1

Beginning on your hands and knees, raise your left leg in a bent position so your thigh is parallel to the floor and your foot points behind you.

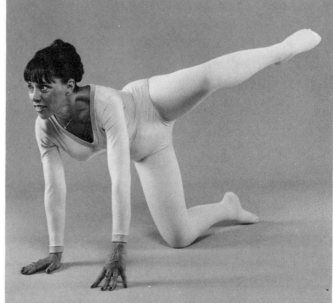

2

Keeping your torso still, raise your left leg higher until you feel your fanny muscles contracting.

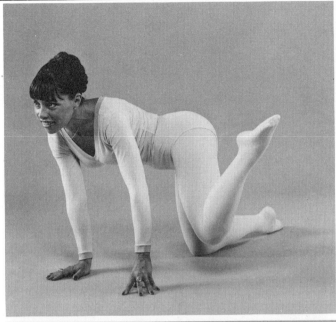

3

Without touching the floor, twist your leg so that the knee faces downward and the toes up.

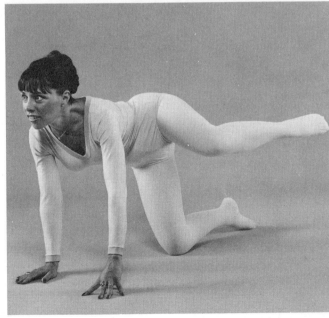

4

Straighten your left leg, then return knee to the floor. Change sides and repeat with your right leg.

Hip Slide

Remember to keep your knees straight and be careful not to arch your lower back. Relax your shoulders and keep your stomach and fanny muscles tightened.

Suzy's Program

Third through seventh week: repeat sequence 8 times

Eighth through twelfth week: repeat sequence 16 times

Thereafter: repeat sequence 24 times

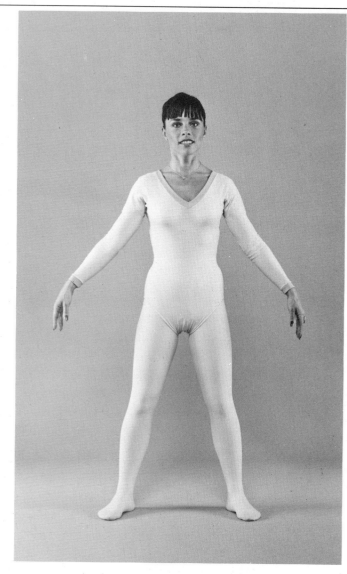

1

Stand straight with your feet apart and your arms raised away from your body. Tighten your stomach and fanny muscles.

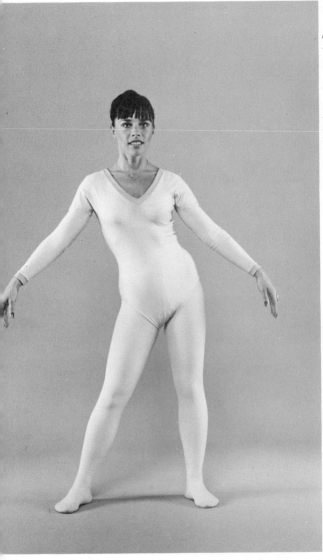

2

Slide your hips as far to the left as you can, keeping your knees straight and your shoulders as still as possible.

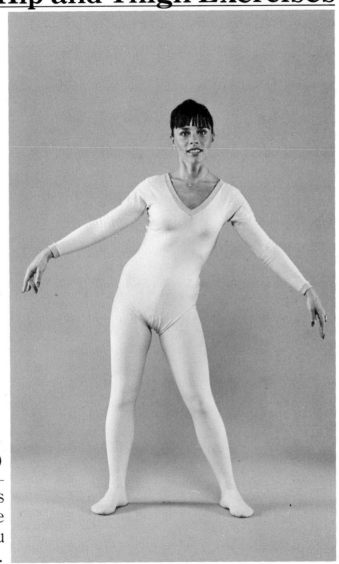

3

Slide your hips as far to the right side as you can.

Hip-up

To help you maintain your balance, keep your stomach and fanny muscles tightened throughout this exercise.

Suzy's Program

Third through seventh week: repeat sequence 4 times

Eighth through twelfth week: repeat sequence 8 times

Thereafter: repeat sequence 12 times

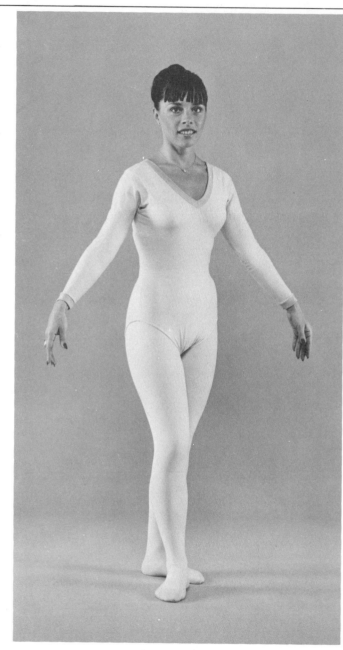

1

Stand straight with your arms raised away from your body. Bend your right knee slightly and place your weight on your left leg.

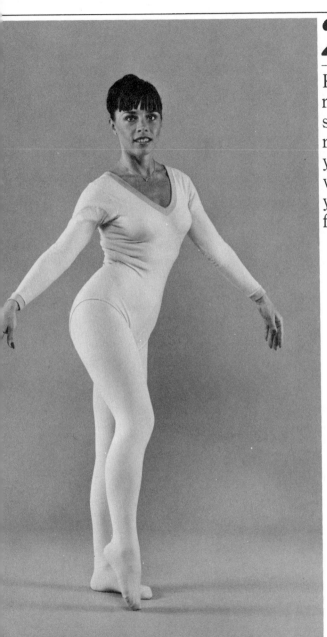

2

Keeping your right knee slightly bent, raise and lower your right hip without lifting your toe off the floor.

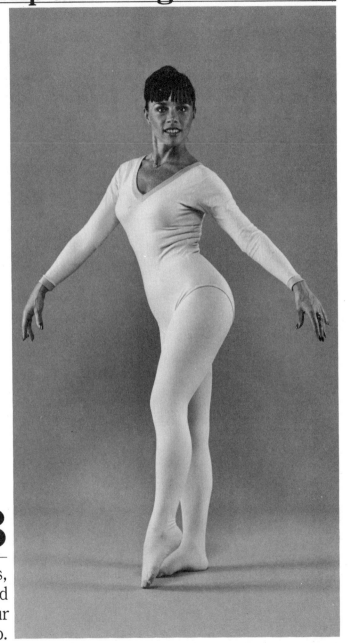

3

Change legs, raising and lowering your left hip.

Back Flat, Leg Lower

Another exercise that is done after as well as during pregnancy. Remember to keep your back flat on the floor as you lower your legs. If your back comes off the floor, you have lowered your legs too far. After a few weeks, however, you will be able to lower your legs a little more with each effort.

Suzy's Program

Third through seventh week: repeat sequence twice

Eighth through twelfth week: repeat sequence 4 times

Thereafter: repeat sequence 8 times

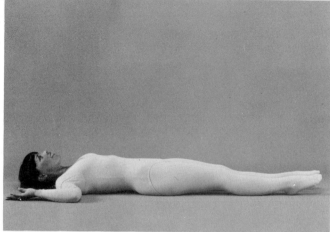

1

Lie on your back, legs straight and feet pointed, with your forearms on the floor parallel to your head.

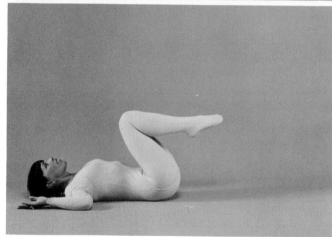

2

Bend your legs and bring them over your chest.

142

3

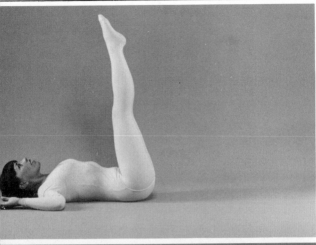

Straighten your knees until your legs are perpendicular to the floor. Keep your legs together, feet pointed, and press your lower back against the floor.

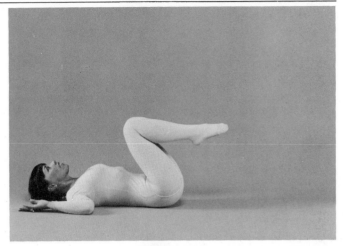

4

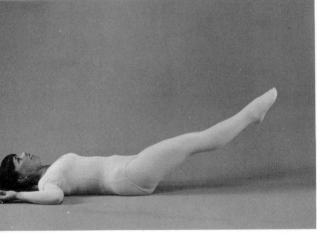

Slowly lower your legs as far as they will go without lifting your lower back off the floor. With your back absolutely flat against the floor, hold this position for 4 seconds.

5

Bring your knees over your chest and rest for 4 seconds. After the final series, bring your knees over your chest and slowly lower your feet to the floor.

Prone Arm Lift

Don't be dismayed if at first you can lift your arms only 1 or 2 inches off the floor. After several weeks of exercising, you will be able to lift them higher. However, be sure that you keep your raised arm straight and close to the side of your head and your body flat on the floor.

Suzy's Program

Third through seventh week: repeat sequence 8 times

Eighth through twelfth week: repeat sequence 12 times

Thereafter: repeat sequence 16 times

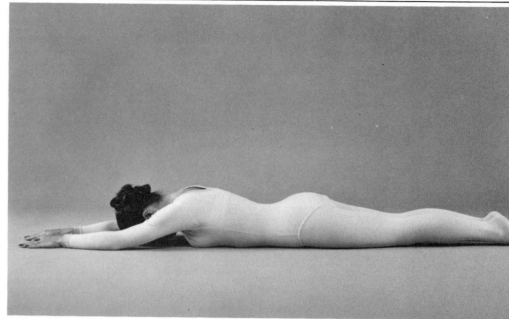

1

Lie on your stomach with your arms stretched out in front.

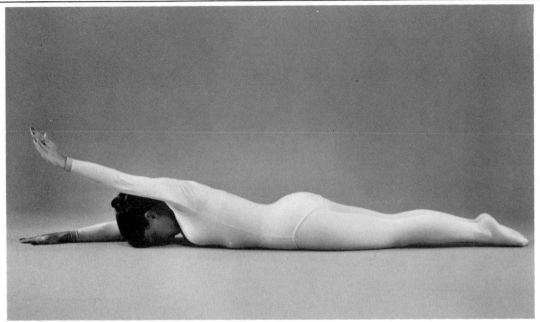

2

Lift your left arm into the air as high as you can, keeping it next to your head. Your torso and forehead should remain on the floor. Lower your left arm, then lift your right arm in the same manner. Don't rock your body from side to side.

Pushing Marbles with Your Nose

This exercise is good not only for your upper back, but for your arms and shoulders as well. It may seem difficult at first, but after a few weeks of exercising, it will become easier.

Suzy's Program

Third through seventh week: repeat sequence 4 times

Eighth through twelfth week: repeat sequence 6 times

Thereafter: repeat sequence 8 times

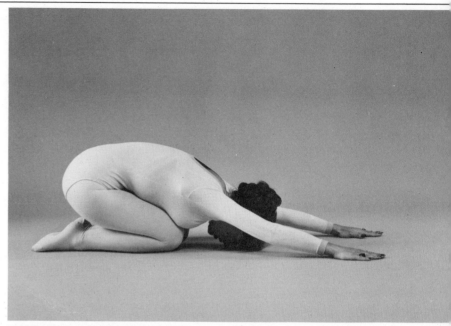

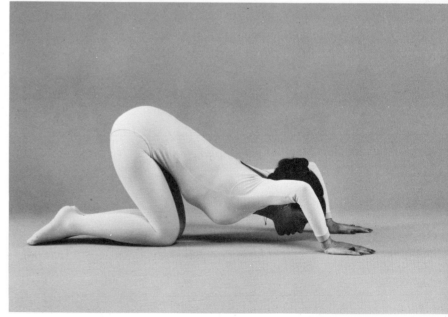

1

Beginning on your hands and knees, stretch your arms out as far as you can in front as you lower your torso to rest on your upper thighs. Keep your fanny as close to your heels as you possibly can.

2

Move your torso forward, keeping your head close to the floor. Bend your elbows so that they stick up into the air.

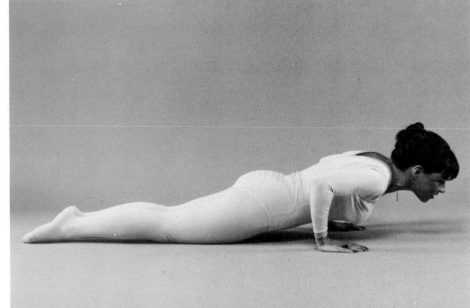

3

Keep pushing your torso forward until it forms a straight line with the floor.

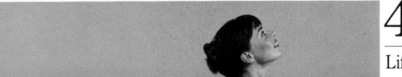

4

Lift your head and straighten your arms, pushing your torso upward. Hold this for 2 seconds. Return to the original position.

Unfolding

The movements in this exercise should be performed as smoothly as possible. It is very good for overall suppleness, as well as upper back strength.

Suzy's Program

Third through seventh week: repeat sequence 4 times

Eighth through twelfth week: repeat sequence 6 times

Thereafter: repeat sequence 8 times

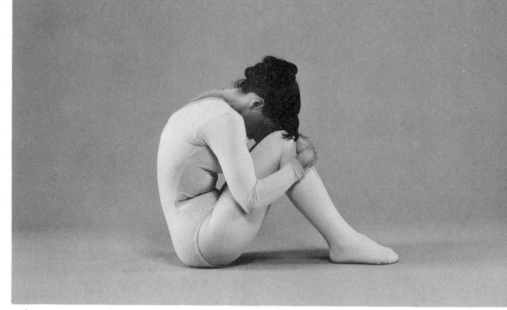

1

Sit with your knees bent and together and your hands clasped around them. Pull in your stomach, round your back, and rest your forehead on your knees.

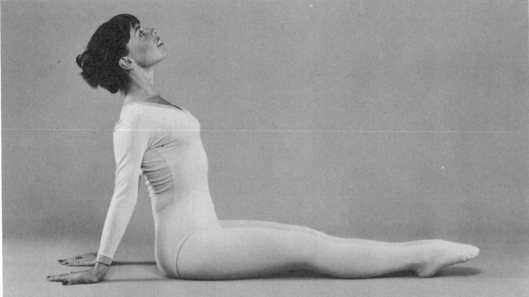

2

Place your hands on the floor behind your fanny and stretch your legs out straight in front of you, feet together and pointed. Arch your back slightly.

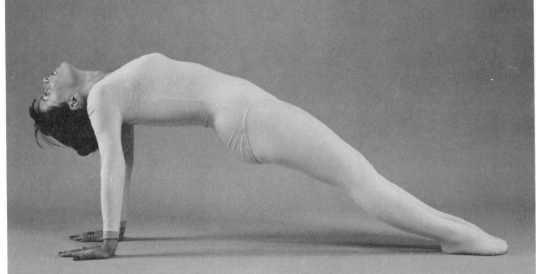

3

Lift your fanny off the floor and straighten your torso. Your body should form a slight arch from feet to chin. Stretch your neck and allow your head to fall back. Hold this position for 4 seconds. Lower your torso and fanny and return to the original sitting position.

Arch and Flatten

This exercise is as effective after as it is during pregnancy to strengthen the lower back muscles while it relieves tension in that region.

Suzy's Program

Third through seventh week: repeat sequence 4 times

Eighth through twelfth week: repeat sequence 6 times

Thereafter: repeat sequence 8 times

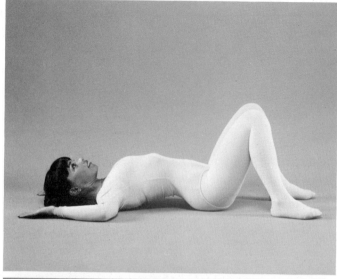

1

Lie on your back with your knees bent and feet flat on the floor. Your forearms are parallel to your head. Arch your lower back so that it is about 2 inches off the floor. Be sure your upper back and fanny remain on the floor. Hold for 2 seconds.

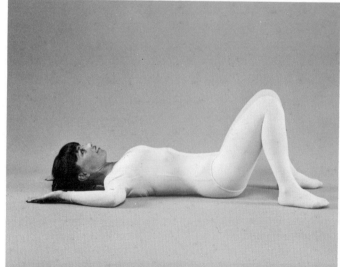

2

Tuck your pelvis under and press your lower back against the floor for 4 seconds, then relax.

The Kitty Stretch

You may find this exercise easier to do after pregnancy than you did during pregnancy. At any time, however, it is effective in reducing muscular tension in the back and shoulder areas.

Suzy's Program

Third through seventh week: repeat sequence 4 times

Eighth through twelfth week: repeat sequence 6 times

Therafter: repeat sequence 8 times

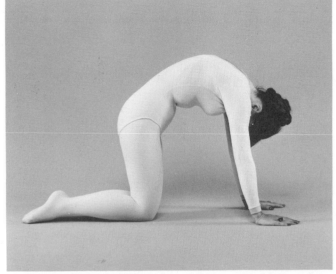

1

Beginning on your hands and knees, round your upper back and lower your head. Tighten your stomach muscles and hold.

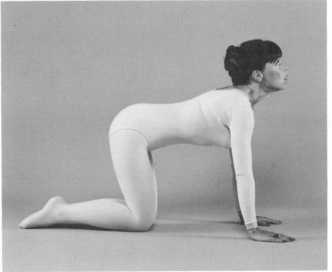

2

In one continuous motion, lift your head stretching and flatten your upper back.

Donkey Kick

When you stretch your leg into the air, do not allow your hip to twist upward. Keep both hips parallel to the floor.

Suzy's Program

Third through seventh week: repeat sequence 4 times

Eighth through twelfth week: repeat sequence 6 times

Thereafter: repeat sequence 8 times

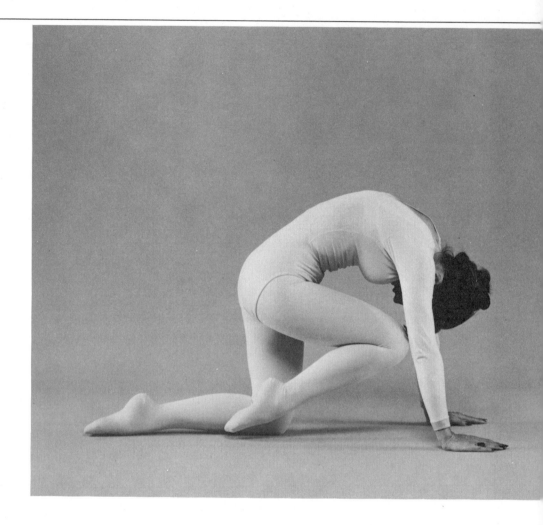

1

Beginning on your hands and knees, lower your head, round your back, and bring your right knee in under your body as close to your head as possible. Pull in your stomach and tighten the muscles in your fanny.

2

In one continuous motion, lift your head and kick your right leg straight back and up behind you. Your raised knee should face the floor and the sole of your foot should face the ceiling. Bend your knee and bring your leg back under your body. Repeat with your left leg.

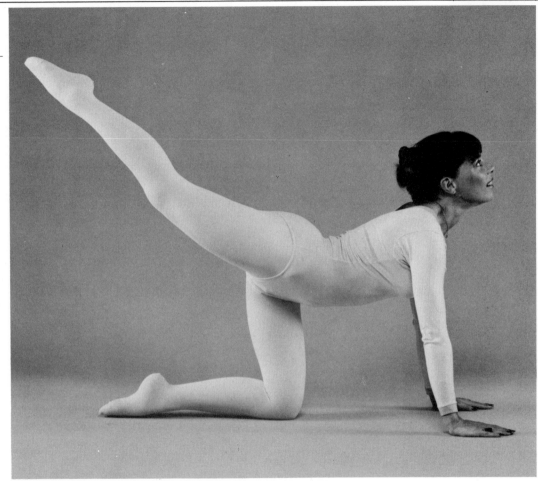

Star Diving

During this exercise, keep your back and legs straight. Do not thrust your head forward or arch your back.

Suzy's Program

Third through seventh week: repeat sequence 4 times

Eighth through twelfth week: repeat sequence 6 times

Thereafter: repeat sequence 8 times

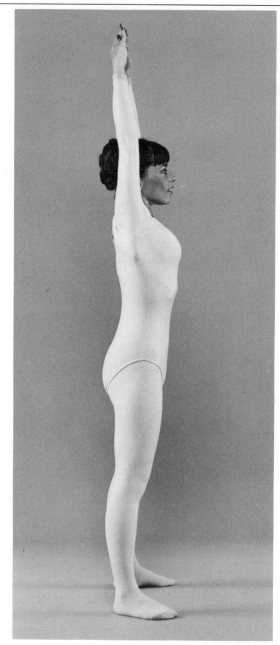

1

Stand straight with your feet apart and your arms extended above your head. Clasp your hands.

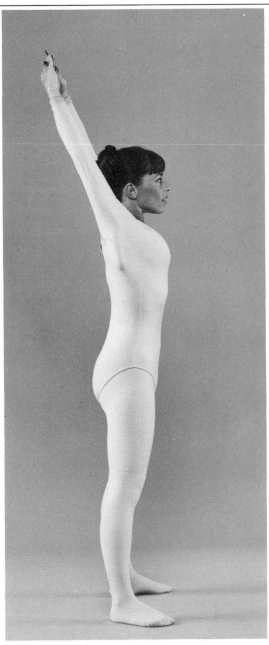

2

Stretch your arms back as far as you can while keeping them and your body straight. Bounce backward 4 times. Return to the original position.

On-knees Push-up

Although simple, this exercise is good for strengthening the arms. Keep your back straight and your knees together.

Suzy's Program

Third through seventh week: repeat sequence 8 times

Eighth through twelfth week: repeat sequence 12 times

Thereafter: repeat sequence 16 times

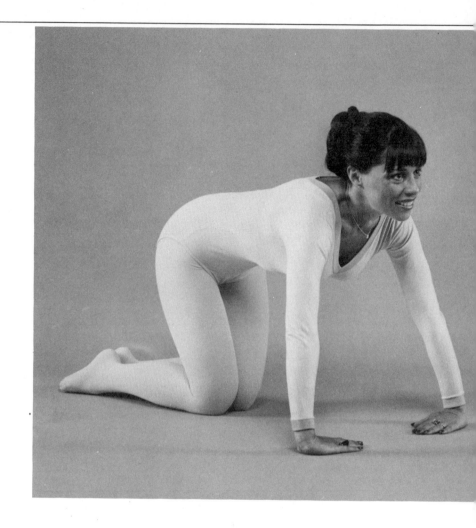

1

Beginning on your hands and knees, place your palms on the floor, hands pointing toward each other.

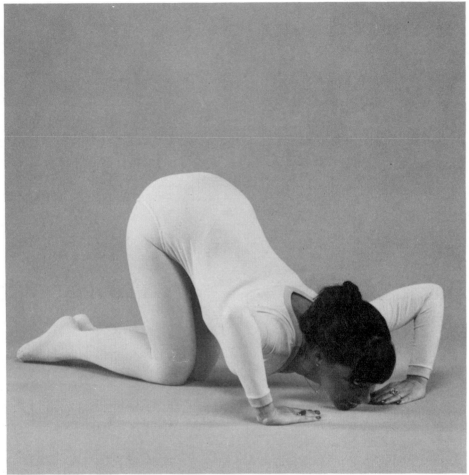

2

Lower your upper torso and your face toward the floor by bending your arms at the elbows. Your chest and chin should just touch the floor. Return to the original position.

Palm Walk

An excellent exercise for your pectoral muscles, it also stretches the backs of your legs. Be sure not to arch your lower back.

Suzy's Program

Third through seventh week: repeat sequence 4 times

Eighth through twelfth week: repeat sequence 6 times,

Thereafter: repeat sequence 8 times

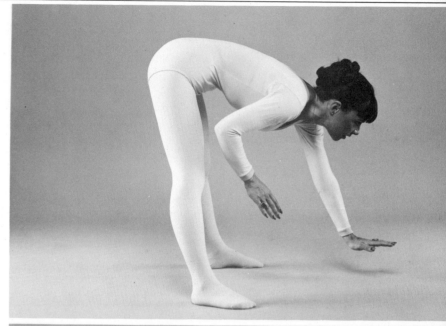

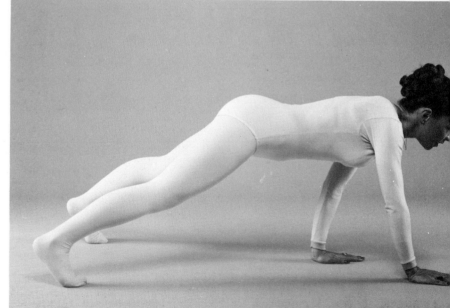

1

Stand with your
legs straight and
feet spread
apart. Bend over
from the waist
and place your
left palm on the
floor.

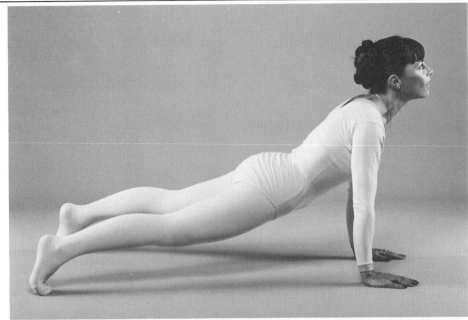

3

Keep your arms
straight as well
as your back.
Tighten your
pectoral muscles
and hold this
position for 4
seconds.

2

Keeping your
legs straight and
your feet in
place, begin to
walk on your
hands, placing
one palm in front
of the other. As
your hands walk
forward, let your
pelvis and torso
drop toward the
floor.

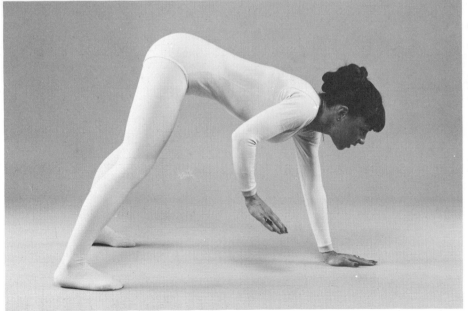

4

Keeping your
legs straight,
walk backward
on your palms to
the original
position.

Midriff Slide

This exercise will not be entirely effective unless you keep the lower part of your body completely still. Watch yourself in a full-length mirror to be sure that only the upper torso moves.

Suzy's Program

Third through seventh week: repeat sequence 4 times

Eighth through twelfth week: repeat sequence 8 times

Thereafter: repeat sequence 12 times

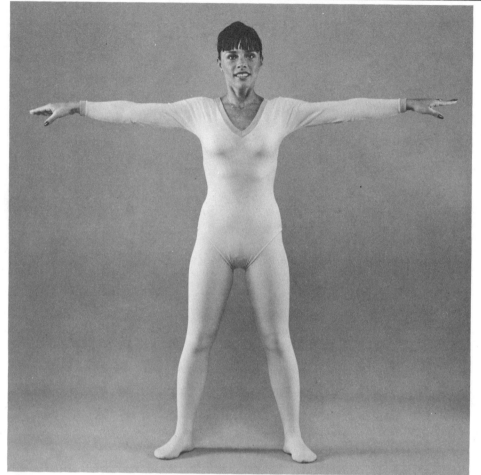

1

Stand straight with your feet apart and your arms stretched out to the sides at shoulder height.

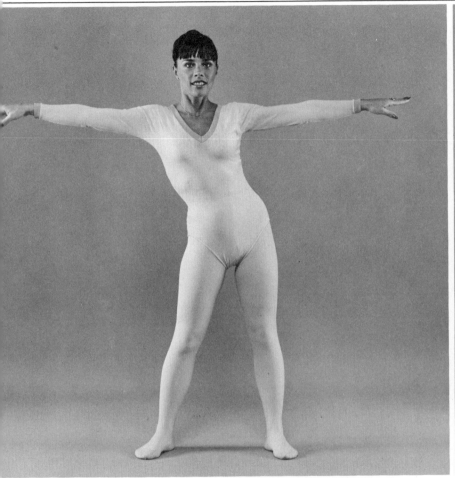

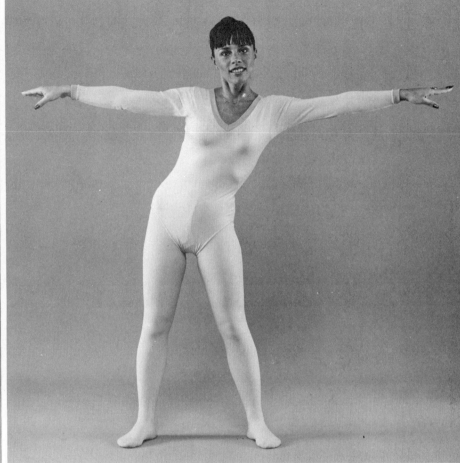

2

Without moving your hips, slide your torso to the right as far as it will go. Keep your shoulders level and your arms straight.

3

Slide your torso to the left, again without moving your hips.

Dipping

This exercise is effective for trimming and toning your waist. Be sure not to arch your lower back or to bend forward at the waist.

Suzy's Program

Third through seventh week: repeat sequence 4 times

Eighth through twelfth week: repeat sequence 6 times

Thereafter: repeat sequence 8 times

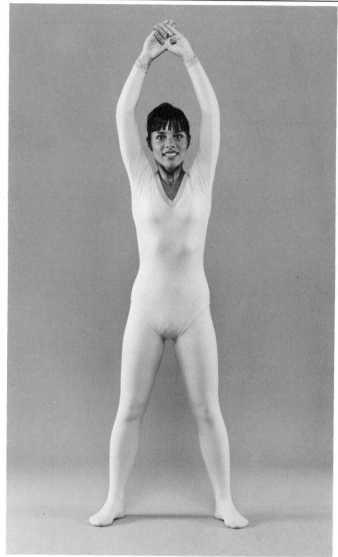

1

Stand straight with your feet apart, arms stretched above your head, and your hands clasped. Tighten your stomach muscles.

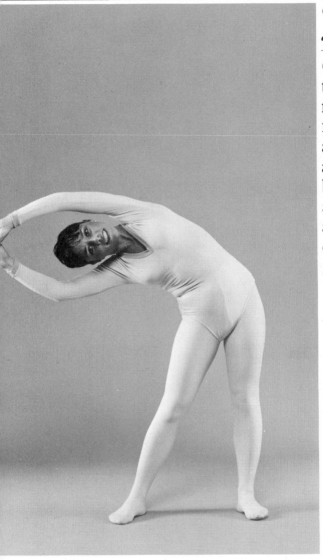

2

Curve your torso to the right, stretching from the waist and without arching your back. Keep your arms straight and your hands clasped. Bounce gently 4 times.

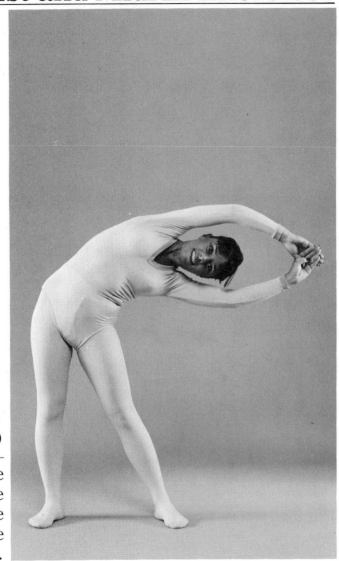

3

In the same manner, curve your torso to the left and bounce gently 4 times.

Propeller Arms

This exercise will help trim the waist and midriff, as well as stretch the backs of legs. If you cannot reach your toes, stretch your arms as far as you comfortably can.

Suzy's Program

Third through seventh week: repeat sequence 8 times

Eighth through twelfth week: repeat sequence 12 times

Thereafter: repeat sequence 16 times

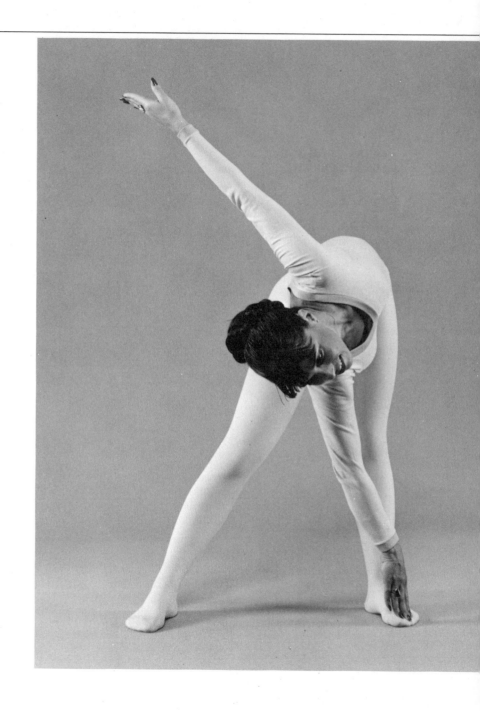

1

With your legs straight and your feet apart, bend forward at your hips. Touch your left foot with your right hand and raise your left arm in the air.

2

Twist your torso to the right, raising your right arm in the air and touching your right foot with your left hand.

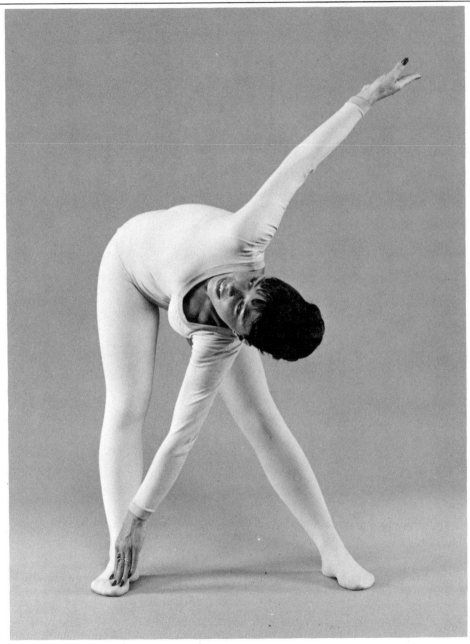

Stick Bend

An excellent exercise for the midriff area. If you do not have a dowel, use a yardstick or broom handle, but be sure your hands are 3 feet apart.

Suzy's Program

Third through seventh week: repeat sequence 4 times

Eighth through twelfth week: repeat sequence 6 times

Thereafter: repeat sequence 8 times

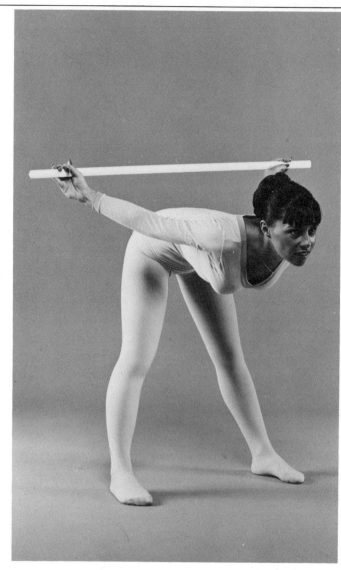

1

Stand with your legs straight and apart, holding a 3-foot dowel with both hands behind you. Your palms should face upward. Without rounding your back, bend forward at the hips until your body is parallel to the floor. Raise your arms slightly, keeping them straight.

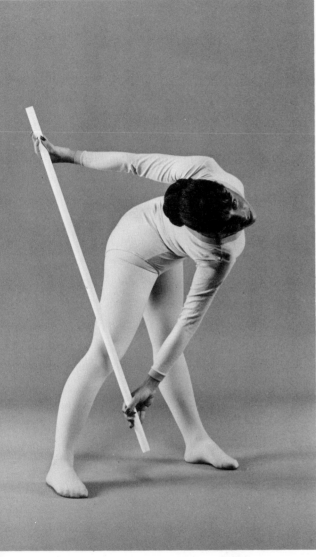

2

Twist your torso to the right, lowering your right shoulder and arm. Your left arm should be stretched backward and your right arm should be in front of your right leg. Do not arch your back.

3

In the same manner, twist your torso to the left, lowering your left shoulder and arm.

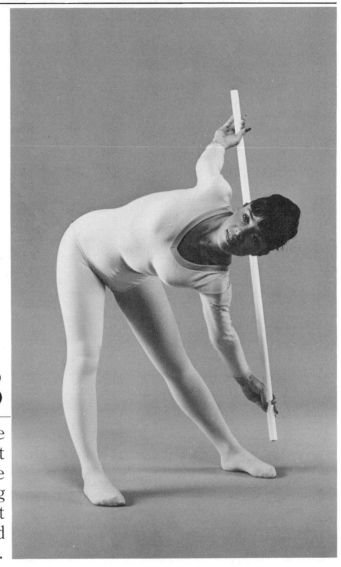

Mime's Walk

Walking is excellent exercise for general fitness. This exercise enables you to walk in place. Raise and lower your heels as slowly as you can.

Suzy's Program

Third through seventh week: repeat sequence 16 times

Thereafter: repeat sequence 24 times

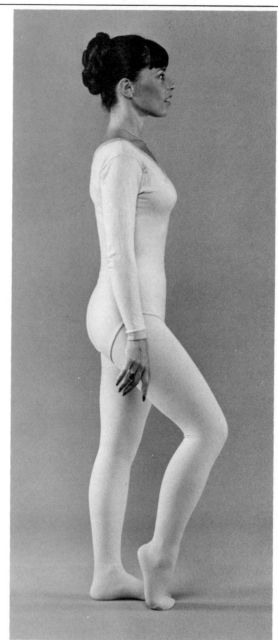

1

Stand with your legs straight, feet together, and arms relaxed at your sides. Tighten your stomach and fanny muscles. Raise your right heel, leaving the ball of your right foot on floor.

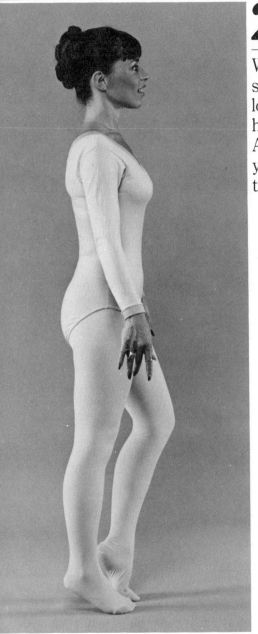

2

With a slow, steady motion, lower your right heel to the floor. As you do so, lift your left heel off the floor.

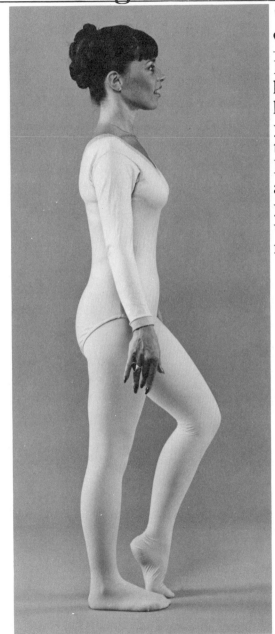

3

Hold your left heel off the floor, leaving the ball of your left foot on the floor. Reverse the action, lowering your left heel while lifting the right heel.

Uphill Knee Bend

This exercise requires considerable balance, so you might want to hold on to the back of a chair or table for support at first. It is important to keep your torso straight.

Suzy's Program

Third through seventh week: repeat sequence 8 times

Eighth through twelfth week: repeat sequence 12 times

Thereafter: repeat sequence 16 times

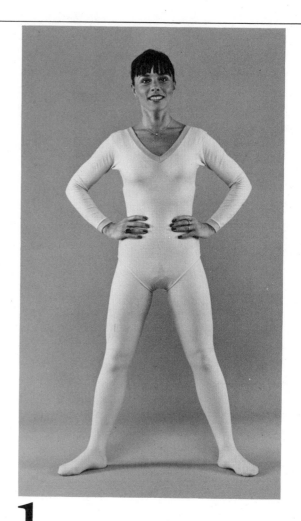

1

Stand with your legs straight, feet apart, and your hands on your hips.

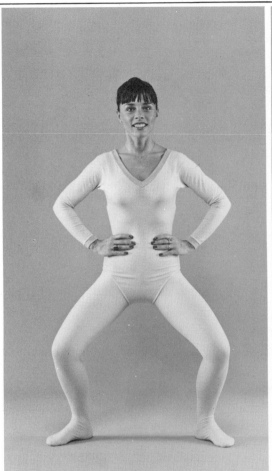

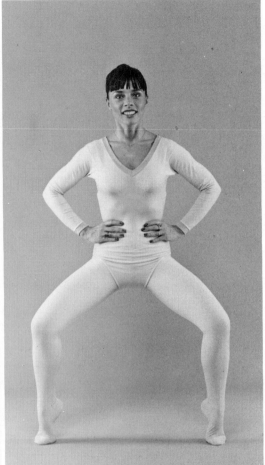

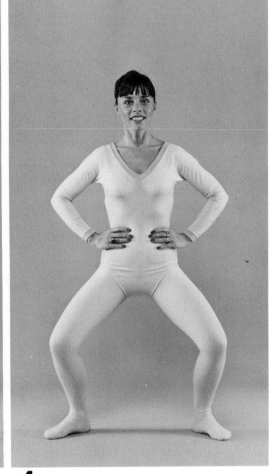

2

Bend your knees and lower your torso about 12 inches, keeping your knees in line with your feet.

3

Without lifting your torso, raise your heels off the floor so that your weight rests on the balls of your feet. Hold for 4 seconds.

4

Then return your heels to the floor.

Plowing

This exercise resembles a series of movements common to beginning skiing lessons. It can help give you strong, flexible legs that do not tire easily. Be sure to keep your feet firmly in place.

Suzy's Program

Third through seventh week: repeat sequence 8 times

Eighth through twelfth week: repeat sequence 12 times

Thereafter: repeat sequence 16 times

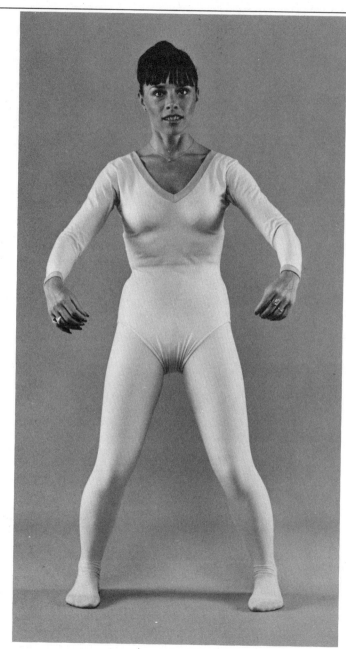

1

Stand with your legs apart, knees slightly bent, and your feet turned in as if pigeon-toed. Your arms should be raised away from your sides. Tuck your pelvis under.

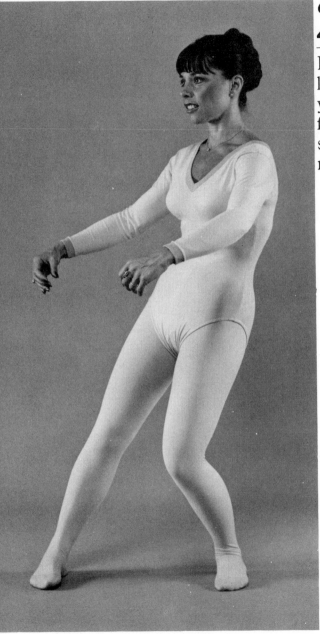

2

Lean on your left leg, twisting your torso to face right as you straighten your right leg.

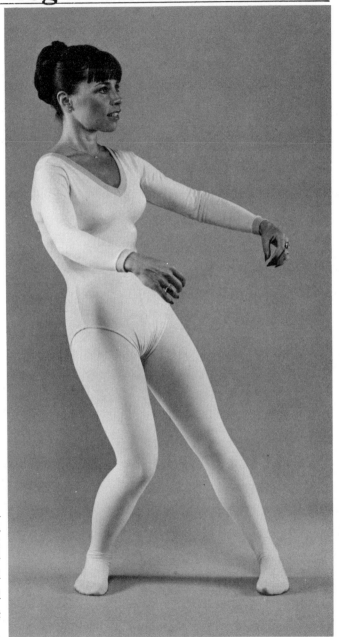

3

Keeping your pelvis tucked under, lean on your right leg in the same manner.

Foot Signatures

By swinging your feet around in a circle while sitting quietly, you can trim your ankles and relax your leg muscles.

Suzy's Program

First week on: repeat exercise as often as you can throughout the day

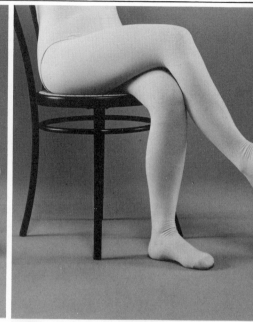

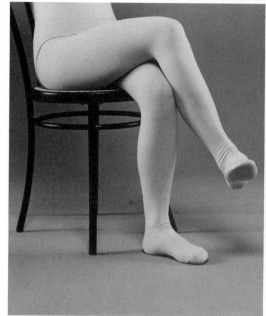

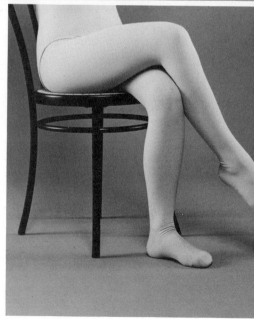

1-3

Sit in a chair and cross one leg over the other. With your raised foot, write your name in imagined script. After 2 weeks, write the entire alphabet with each foot.

Flex That Foot

When your toes are curled, your weight should rest on the outsides of your feet. This exercise is good for stretching your Achilles tendons and preventing cramps in your lower legs.

Suzy's Program

Third through seventh week: repeat sequence 8 times

Eighth through twelfth week: repeat sequence 12 times

Thereafter: repeat sequence 16 times

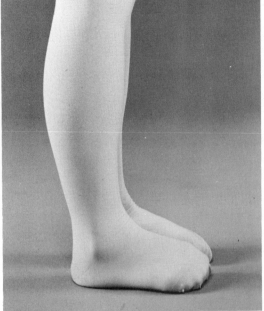

1

Stand with your feet together and legs straight. Curl your toes under as if digging them into a sandy beach. Hold this position for 2 seconds.

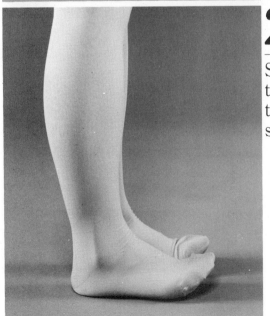

2

Stretch your toes up toward your body and hold that position for 2 seconds.

Up and Down

This exercise strengthens your ankles, relieves tension in the calf muscles, and helps your balance.

Suzy's Program

Third through seventh week: repeat sequence 4 times

Eighth through twelfth week: repeat sequence 6 times

Thereafter: repeat sequence 8 times

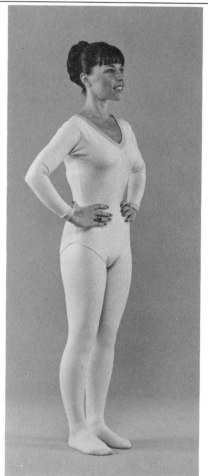

1

Stand with your legs straight, feet together, and your hands on your hips. Tighten your stomach and fanny muscles.

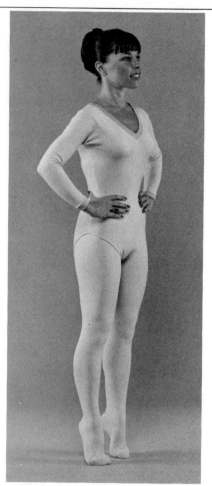

2

Rise slowly onto the balls of your feet and hold this position for 4 seconds. Then lower your heels to the floor.

1

Jumping Rope

Although primarily a cardio-vascular exercise, jumping rope is excellent for toning and strengthening your legs.

Suzy's Program

Third through seventh week: 10 to 30 seconds of jumping

Eighth through twelfth week: 1 to 2 minutes of jumping

Thereafter: 3 minutes of jumping

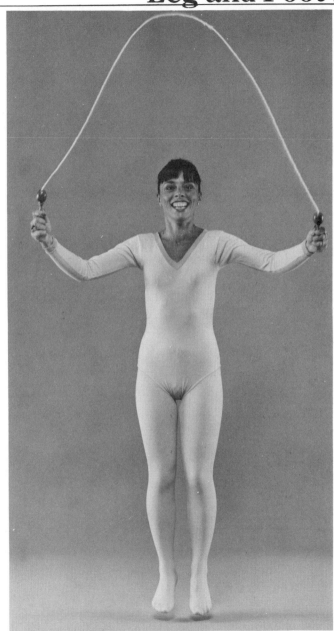

Jump rope with your feet a few inches apart and knees bent slightly. Start with 10 seconds a day and work up to 3 minutes after 12 weeks of regular jumping.

Infant
Starters

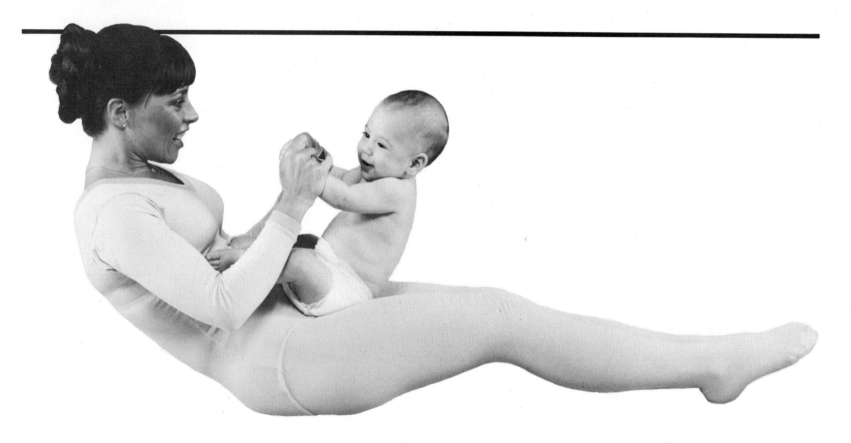

Many parents once looked upon babies merely as objects to be hugged, bathed, fed, and diapered. And that was about the extent of it. However, when infant-exercise programs became generally accepted, parents found that new ways had been opened for communication with their babies. Through exercise, parents and babies are able to participate in an active form of intimacy that is warm, loving, and healthful. It is so much more beneficial for a baby to have its parents manipulate its arms and legs than it is for the baby to be left in a crib, where only listlessness and sleep are natural. When a baby is exercised, the baby's face lights up with pleasure—eyes twinkle, lips smile, and the baby coos with pleasure. That is an infant's way of expressing happiness—and the parent is gratified.

A baby who has two pleasurable exercise sessions each day will experience a loving interaction with mommy and daddy nearly from birth onward. And that interaction will have far more positive results than a schedule that includes only feeding, burping, diapering, and napping.

Exercises should be started in infancy and done regularly throughout the first three years of a child's life. Of course, exercises are an important lifelong activity, but the first three years of life are of crucial importance. It is during that time that 50 percent of a child's physical and intellectual potential is formed.

The value of infant exercise has been carefully documented at a number of leading research centers, including the Harvard Pre-School Project under the direction of Dr. Burton L. White and at the University of Chicago by Dr. Benjamin S. Bloom. At the Institute for the Care of Mother and Child in Czechoslovakia, Dr. Jaroslav Koch began a program of exercise for a large number of infants who were only four weeks old. Children in the program learned to talk earlier, had better appetites, slept more soundly, and experienced a greater acceleration in their motor development than children who hadn't been exercised. At Suzy Prudden Studios in New York City, infant exercise programs were begun as early as 1966, prior to any research studies. And the results were exactly the same.

179

Since then, many babies have been through the infant exercise program at the studio.

Infant exercises accelerate motor development, coordination and agility, increasing flexibility and strength. Exercised infants who continue with our program into the toddler age begin to understand their limitations, have self-confidence, and are not timid about accepting new challenges.

The exercises that follow are for the first eight months of your baby's life and help provide a firm foundation for an ongoing program of physical fitness. They are an enjoyable activity that will establish firm bonds between parent and child. Baby will grow to look forward to these sessions, and you will have established the groundwork upon which to build a relationship of intimacy, trust, and affection.

General rules you should follow before you exercise your baby as well as during the actual exercise sessions:

- Ask your pediatrician if there are any exercises your baby should not do; make sure that it is all right to begin the overall exercise program.
- Always place your baby on a soft surface, such as a blanket that is folded into a cushion on the floor. Never exercise the baby on a table, chair, or other high object, because the baby could accidentally fall.
- You should try to exercise your baby twice each day. However, if your baby cries, stop. The exercises should always be an enjoyable and positive experience.
- Make sure that your baby is physically comfortable. A diaper is adequate clothing, but only if your baby is not lying in a draft.
- Frequently check baby's face for reactions while doing the exercises. A smile means that everything is going well.
- Never exercise when your baby is hungry or tired; and never exercise right after your baby has finished eating or immediately after awakening.
- Never do too much with a baby—do not try to set any records. Also, do not force limbs or torso to bend in ways they were not meant to bend.

- Frequently interrupt the exercise sessions with hugs and kisses. Always talk to your baby, offering praise and signs of love and affection.
- An exercise session should never last longer than 20 minutes. If baby loses interest or starts to fret, end the session with a hug.

Baby Push-ups

It may take several attempts before your baby knows to push up with its arms. In time, however, the baby will use its arms to hold head and chest off the floor throughout this exercise. Be sure to support your baby's torso and hips; never hold just the thighs.

Suzy's Program

Second through third month:
repeat sequence 4 times

Fourth through fifth month:
repeat sequence 6 times

Sixth through eighth month:
repeat sequence 8 times

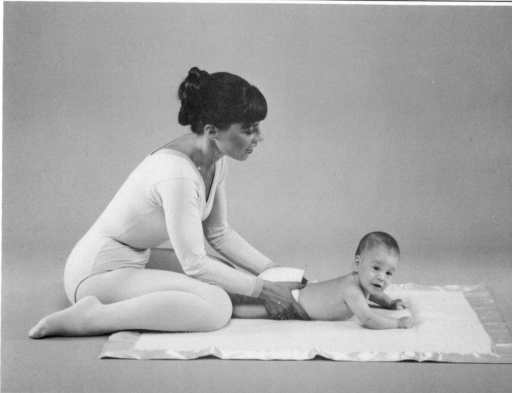

1

Place your baby on its stomach with arms out in front. Gently, but firmly, hold your baby by the hips, stomach, and chest. As your baby becomes stronger, hold only the hips and stomach, then just the hips.

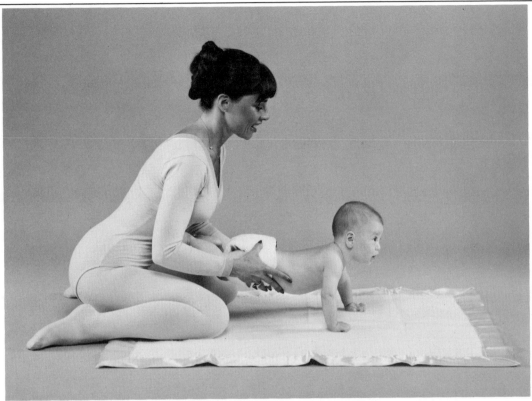

2

Slowly lift your baby so that its torso is raised no higher than the length of its arms. Your baby's arms will usually extend themselves, providing additional support and balance. Then slowly lower your baby's torso to the floor and rest there for 2 seconds before repeating.

Hands-up

This exercise should be started only when your baby is capable of holding its head in an upright position without support.

Suzy's Program

Second through third month: repeat sequence 4 times

Fourth through fifth month: repeat sequence 6 times

Sixth through eighth month: repeat sequence 8 times

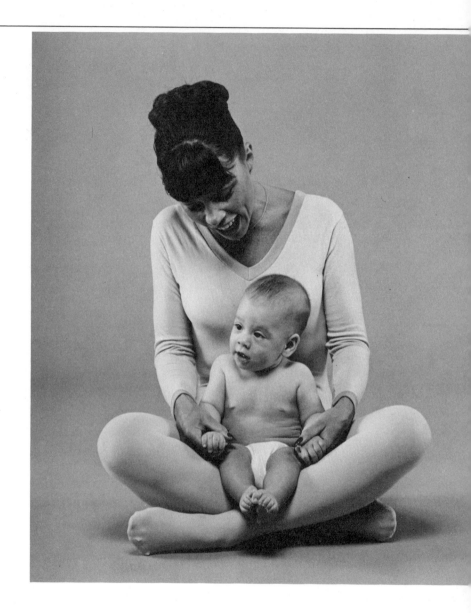

1

Sit on the floor with your
legs crossed and place
your baby in your lap. You
and baby should be facing
in the same direction.
Have your baby clasp your
index fingers, then wrap
your baby's wrists with
your thumbs and fingers.

2

Slowly raise your baby's
arms above its head.
Gently stretch them into a
straight position. Then
lower your baby's arms.
Do not allow your baby to
fall forward when lowering
the arms.

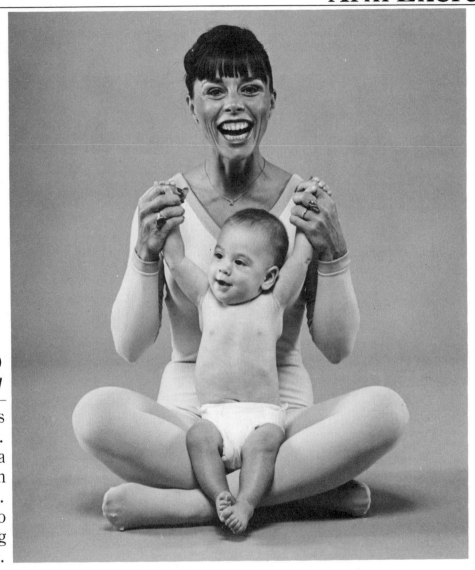

Gentle Arm Twist

A simple but good exercise to strengthen the muscles in your baby's upper arms.

Suzy's Program

Second through third month: repeat sequence 4 times

Fourth through fifth month: repeat sequence 6 times

Sixth through eighth month: repeat sequence 8 times

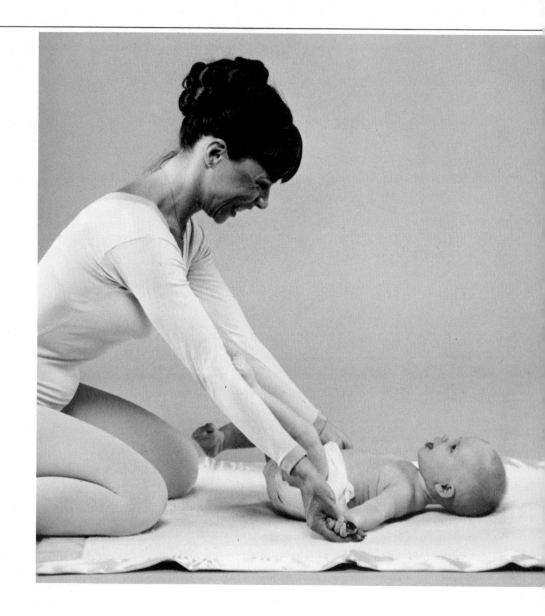

1

Place your baby on its back and gently hold each hand. Turn each of your baby's arms out so that the palms face upward.

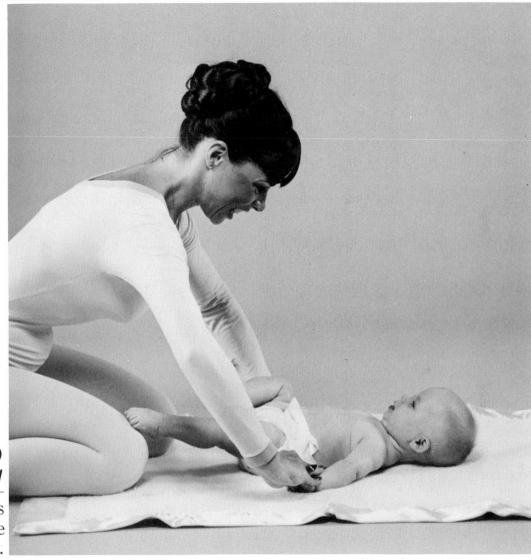

2

Turn your baby's arms so that the palms face downward.

Alternate Arm Stretch

An exercise that your baby will enjoy, it helps strengthen the baby's arms, shoulders, and chest. Keep the arm movements steady and smooth.

Suzy's Program

Second through third month: repeat sequence 4 times

Fourth through fifth month: repeat sequence 6 times

Sixth through eighth month: repeat sequence 8 times

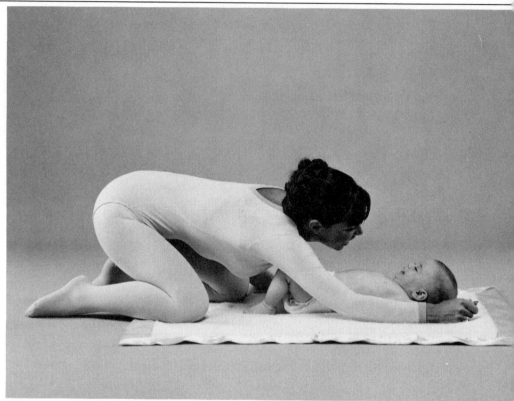

1

Place your baby on its back. Have your baby clasp your thumbs, then wrap your fingers around its hands. Hold your baby's left arm above its head, while you bring baby's right arm straight down by its side.

188

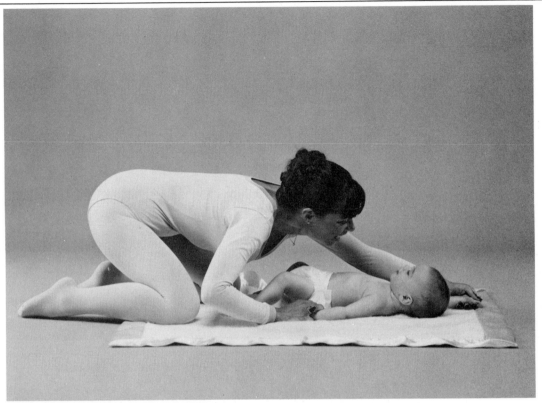

2

Reverse the arms,
stretching the right one
above its head and the left
down by its side.

Bird's-eye View

The first few times you do this exercise, have your spouse place your baby's hands on the floor while you lower its torso to the floor. In a very short time, your baby will learn to reach for the floor for support.

Suzy's Program

Second through third month: repeat sequence twice, lifting baby 6 inches off the floor

Fourth through fifth month: repeat sequence 4 times, lifting baby 2 feet off the floor

Sixth through eighth month: repeat sequence 6 times, lifting baby 3 feet off the floor

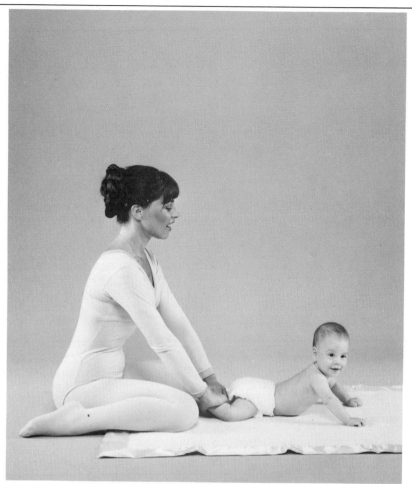

1

Place your baby on its stomach. Firmly grasp your baby's legs.

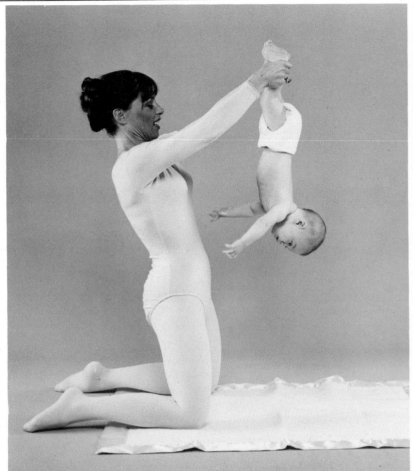

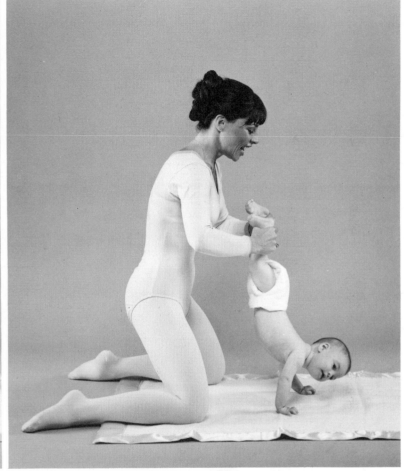

2

Gently and slowly lift your baby off the floor. Hold your baby upside down for 3 seconds. Your baby will arch its lower back, developing strong muscles that are necessary for good posture.

3

Slowly lower your baby to the original position. Do not be frightened if at first your baby's face touches the floor before its chest.

191

Flying

This enjoyable exercise makes most babies smile. It helps develop strong back muscles in your baby and a feeling of trust toward the parent. The baby's self-confidence is also enhanced as a result of this exercise.

Suzy's Program

Second through third month: repeat sequence 4 times

Fourth through fifth month: repeat sequence 6 times

Sixth through eighth month: repeat sequence 8 times

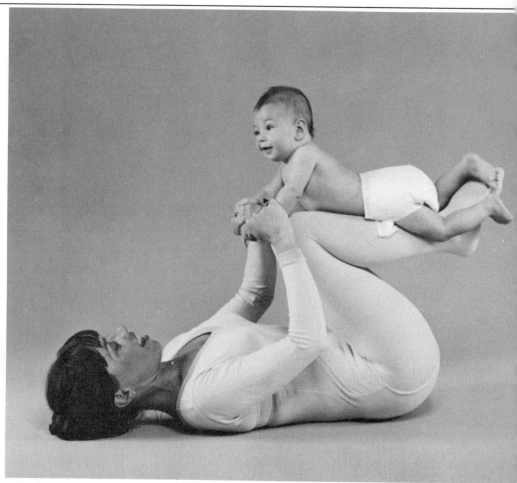

1

Lie flat on your back with your legs raised and bent so that your calves are parallel to the floor. Carefully place your baby on your shins; its chest should be on your knees. Hold your baby's hands.

2

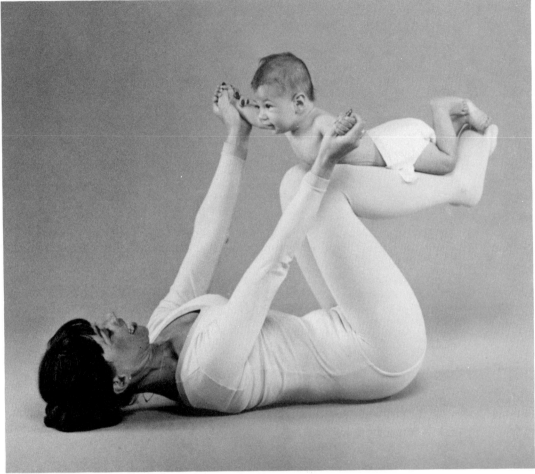

While you raise your feet slightly so that your baby's legs are higher than its chest, gently stretch your baby's arms out to the side. Your baby should be able to lift its own head and arch its back. Hold this position for 4 seconds. While you lower your legs to the original position, bring your baby's hands in to meet in front of your knees.

Back Over

While doing this exercise be especially careful not to lift your baby's legs too far or your baby may experience discomfort. This exercise requires practice and patience, but it will effectively strengthen and stretch your baby's back muscles.

Suzy's Program

Second through third month: repeat sequence 4 times

Fourth through fifth month: repeat sequence 6 times

Sixth through eighth month: repeat sequence 8 times

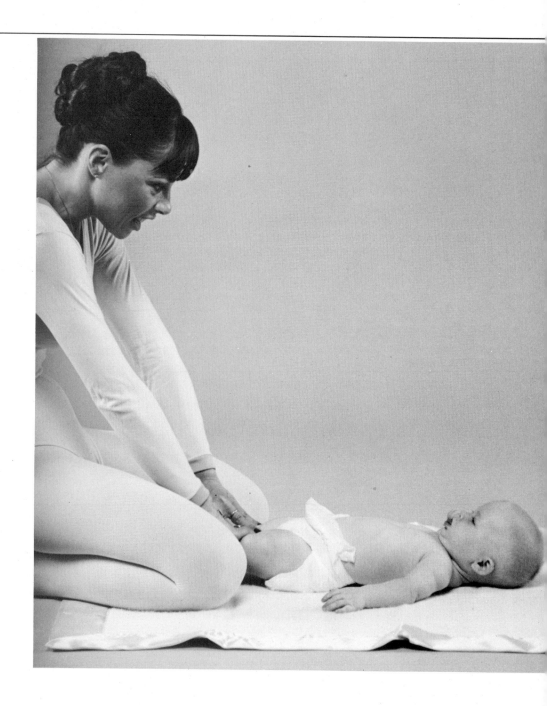

1

Place your baby on its back. Hold each of your baby's legs with your fingers wrapped around the thighs and your thumbs on the calves.

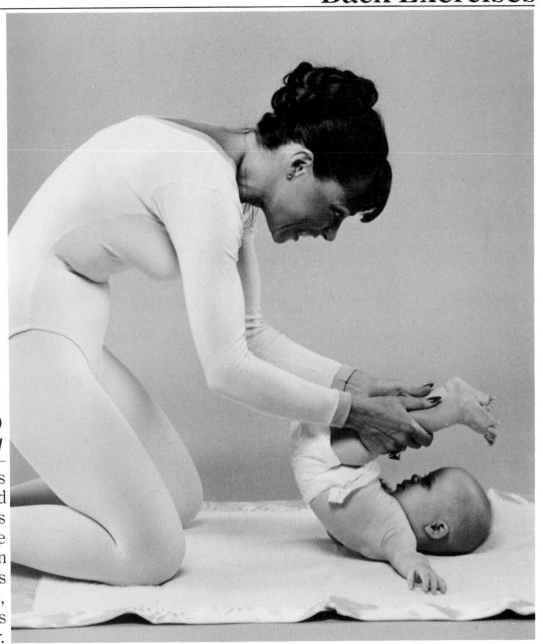

2

Slowly lift your baby's legs over its stomach and chest so that the baby's fanny is raised off the floor and its weight is on its upper back. Hold this position for 2 seconds, then lower your baby's legs to the floor.

Salute

This exercise shouldn't be started until your baby is 3 or 4 months old. It is excellent for developing your baby's back muscles and self-confidence.

Suzy's Program

From time you start: repeat sequence twice

Four weeks later: repeat sequence 4 times

Thereafter: repeat sequence 6 times

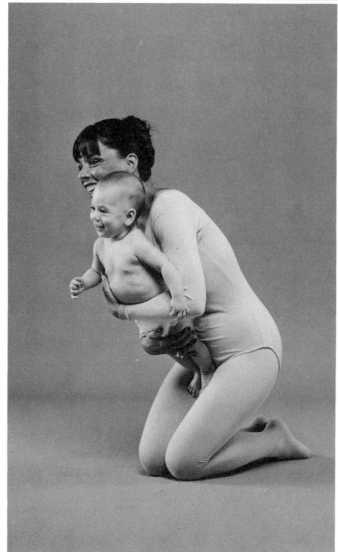

1

Kneeling, bend at the waist, hug your baby against your chest, and place your baby's feet on your thighs. Hold your baby with one arm around the stomach and the other arm around the upper thighs.

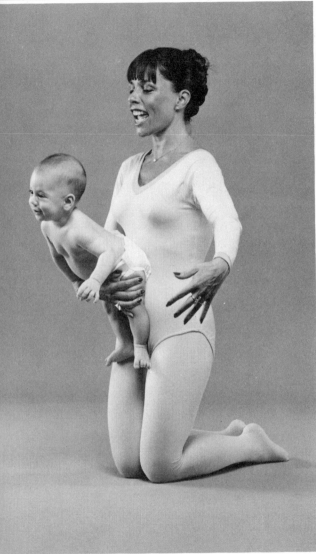

2

Without pulling your baby up with you, release the hand holding the baby's stomach and slowly straighten your body so that your baby is at a 45-degree angle to your body.

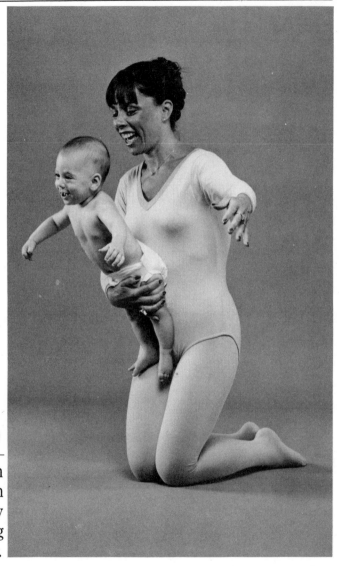

3

Hold this position for 2 seconds, then lower your body and gently hug your baby.

Pectoral Stretch

This is an extremely simple exercise, but one that is very good for strengthening and stretching your baby's pectoral muscles.

Suzy's Program

Second through third month: repeat sequence 6 times

Fourth through fifth month: repeat sequence 8 times

Sixth through eighth month: repeat sequence 12 times

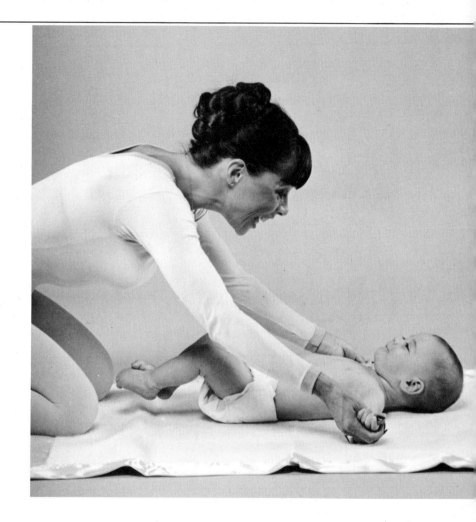

1

Place your baby on its back. Have your baby clasp your thumbs, then wrap your fingers around the baby's hands. Stretch your baby's arms out to the side at shoulder height.

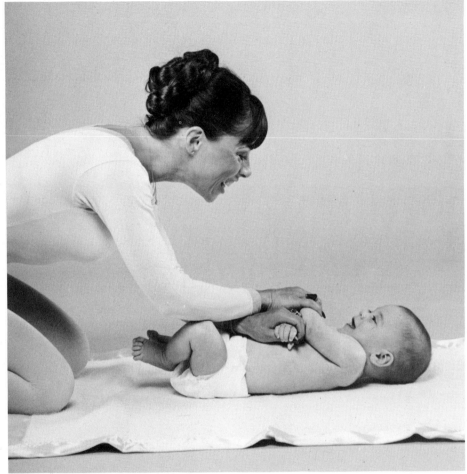

2

Then cross your baby's arms over its chest.

Arm Stretch and Alternating Stretch

Babies' arms have a tendency to remain bent during their early months of life. This exercise helps stretch those otherwise contracted muscles.

Suzy's Program

Second through third month:
steps 1-2, 4 times; steps 3-4, 8 times

Fourth through fifth month:
steps 1-2, 6 times; steps 3-4, 12 times

Sixth through eighth month:
steps 1-2, 8 times; steps 3-4, 12 times

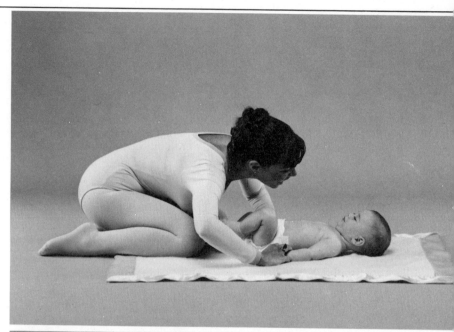

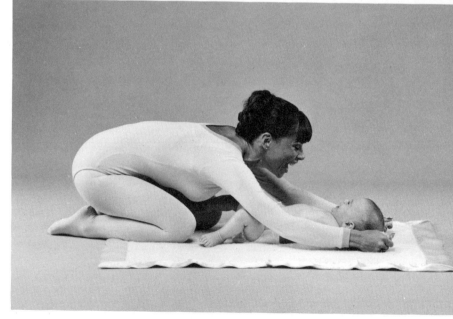

1

Place your baby on its back. Have your baby clasp your thumbs, then wrap your fingers around your baby's hands.

2

Raise your baby's arms straight above its head, then lower them to the baby's sides.

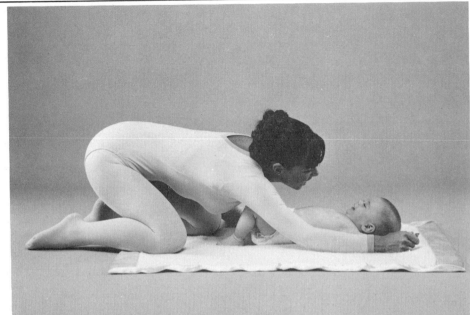

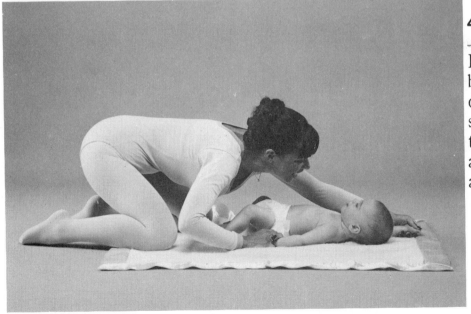

3

While keeping your baby's right arm at its right side, raise the baby's left arm above its head.

4

Bring your baby's left arm down to the left side as you raise the baby's right arm straight above its head.

Sitting Crossover

A variation of Hands-up, this exercise stretches and strengthens your baby's chest and upper back muscles.

Suzy's Program

Second through third month: repeat sequence 4 times

Fourth through fifth month: repeat sequence 6 times

Sixth through eighth month: repeat sequence 8 times

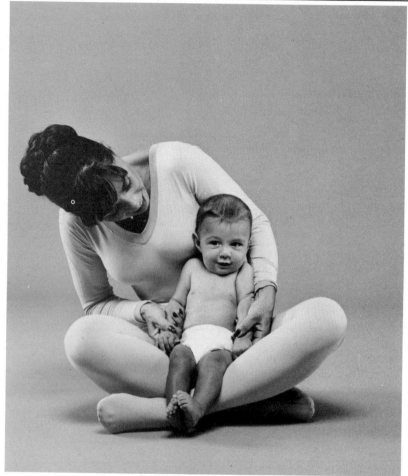

1

Sit on the floor with your legs crossed and place your baby in your lap. You and baby should face the same direction. Have your baby clasp your index fingers, then wrap your fingers around your baby's hands and wrists.

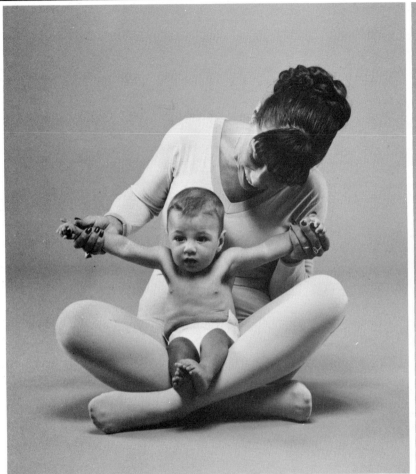

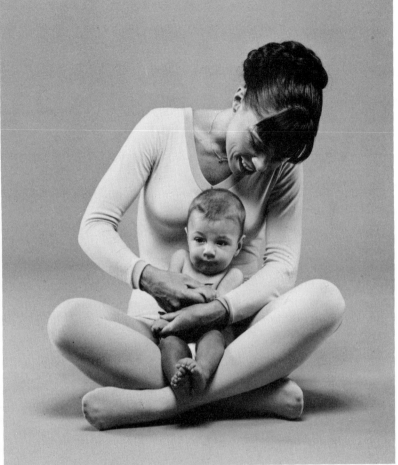

2

Stretch your baby's arms
out to the sides at
shoulder height.

3

Then bring your baby's
arms in and across its
chest.

Baby's Bicycle

Even babies have their version of the bicycle exercise! It is excellent for strengthening your baby's stomach muscles, as well as keeping legs limber and flexible.

Suzy's Program

Second through third month: repeat sequence once

Fourth through fifth month: repeat sequence twice

Sixth through eighth month: repeat sequence 3 times

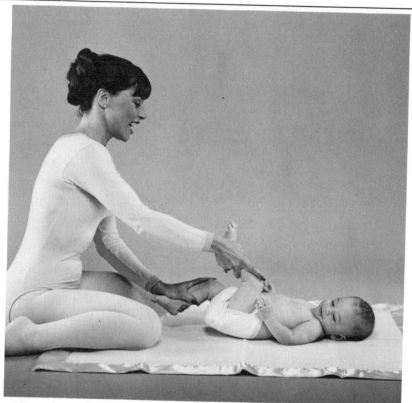

1

Place your baby on its back and grasp both legs in your hands.

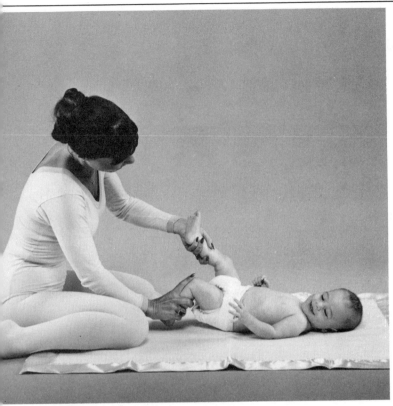

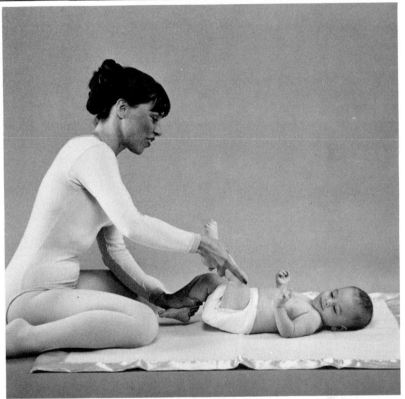

2

Rotate your baby's legs as
if your baby were riding a
bicycle. Make six
rotations.

3

Rotate your baby's legs six
times in the other
direction as if your baby
were riding a bicycle
backwards.

Scissors

While strengthening your baby's stomach muscles, this exercise helps keep legs strong and flexible. As always, keep your movements smooth and gentle.

Suzy's Program

Second through third month:
repeat sequence 6 times

Fourth through fifth month:
repeat sequence 8 times

Sixth through eighth month:
repeat sequence 12 times

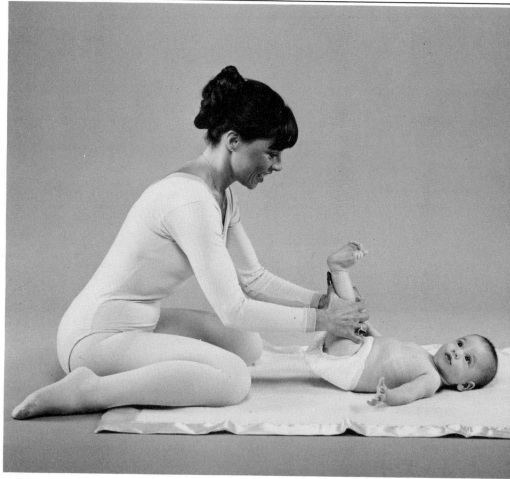

1

Place your baby on its back and clasp the baby's legs at the knees. Raise both legs until they are perpendicular to the floor.

Your baby's legs should be together and as straight as possible and its back flat on the floor.

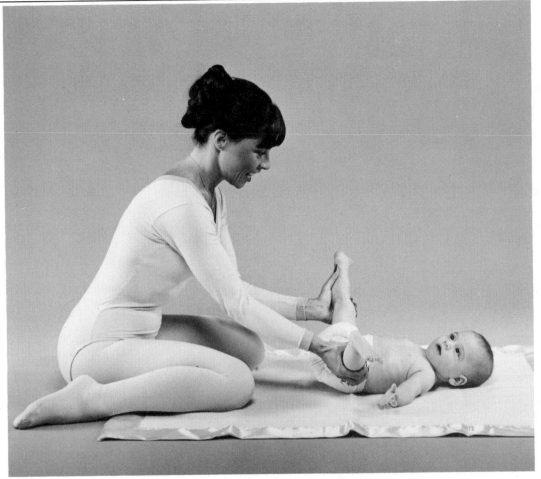

2

Slowly separate your baby's legs, lowering them as far as they can comfortably go to each side. Return to the original position.

The Sit-up

During this exercise do not let your baby's head fall backward. If your baby is unable to hold its head up, place one of your hands behind its head for support. After several weeks, your baby will be able to sit up and lie down without your support behind its head.

Suzy's Program

Second through third month:
repeat sequence 4 times

Fourth through fifth month:
repeat sequence 6 times

Sixth through eighth month:
repeat sequence 8 times

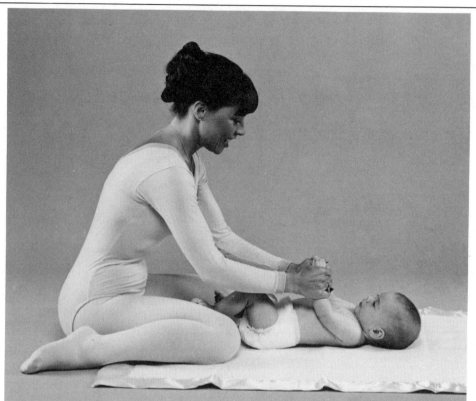

1

Place your baby on its back. Have your baby clasp your thumbs, then wrap your fingers around the baby's hands.

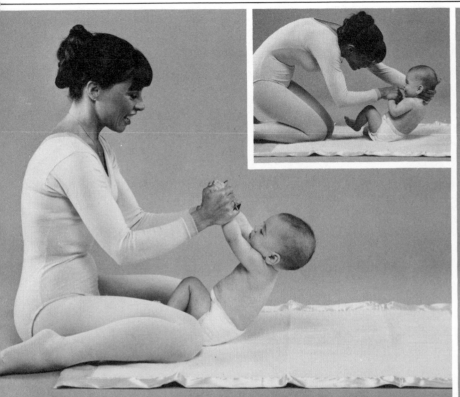

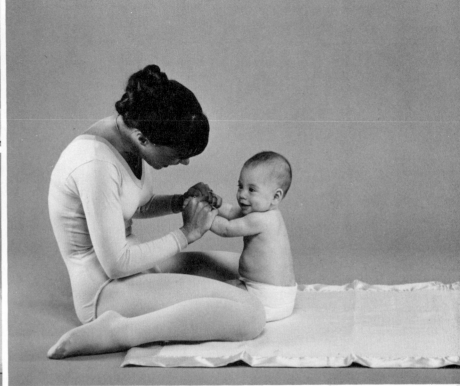

2

Very gently and smoothly, pull your baby up into a sitting position. If you must support your baby's head, place one of your hands behind it and use your other to clasp the baby's hands.

3

Pull your baby into a full sitting position. Then slowly lower the baby to its original supine position, supporting your baby's head if necessary.

Sit-ups for Two

This exercise is more like a game than an exercise. For your baby it provides the same kind of fun as a rocking horse or being bounced on a parent's knee. For the mother, it helps to strengthen her stomach muscles.

Suzy's Program

Second through third month: repeat sequence twice

Fourth through fifth month: repeat sequence 4 times

Sixth through eighth month: repeat sequence 8 times

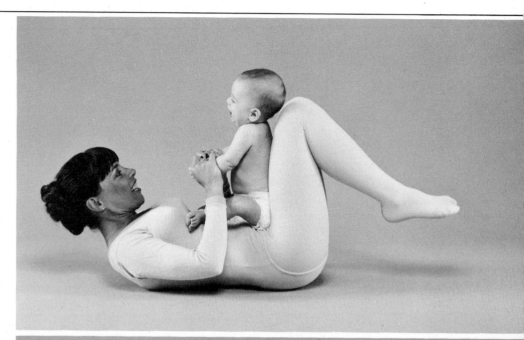

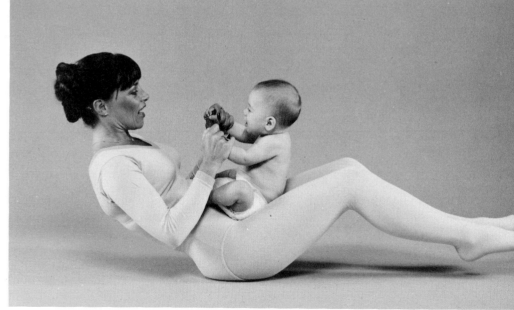

1

Lie on your back with your knees bent and feet flat on the floor. Place your baby on your stomach with its back resting against your thighs. Raise your feet slightly off the floor to support your baby's back. Have your baby clasp your thumbs, then wrap your fingers around your baby's hands.

2

Slowly lower your legs so that they no longer support your baby's back.

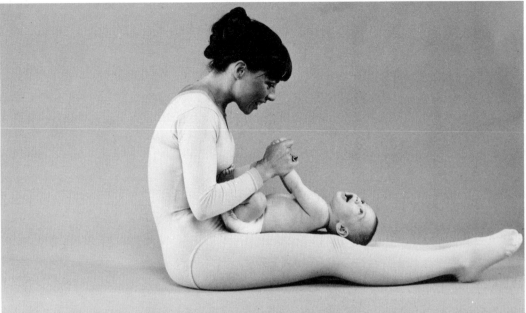

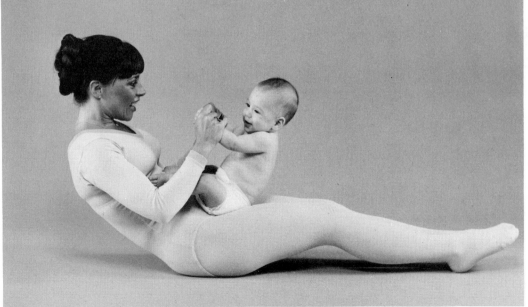

3

Raise your torso into a sitting position and lower your baby so that it lies flat on your straight legs.

4

Slowly round your back and return to your original position, gently pulling your baby into a sitting position, supporting its back with your thighs.

Knee Bends

This is one of the most effective exercises for straightening, stretching, and strengthening your baby's legs. Many mothers have found this exercise relieves crankiness in their babies.

Suzy's Program

Second through third month:
repeat sequence 8 times

Fourth through fifth month:
repeat sequence 12 times

Sixth through eighth month:
repeat sequence 16 times

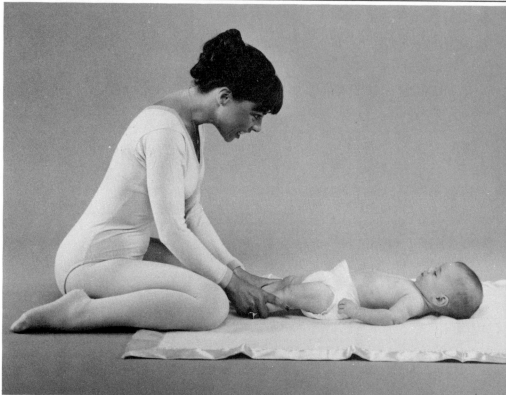

1

Place your baby on its back. Clasp of your baby's legs and hold them so that they are straight.

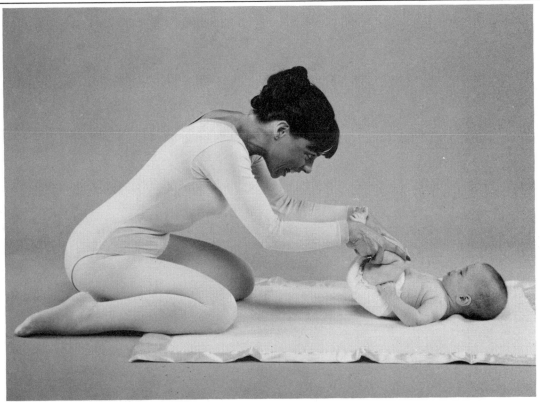

2

Bend your baby's knees
over its chest, then
straighten them to the
original position.

Alternate Knee Bends

This exercise offers the same benefits as Knee Bends, and also it helps improve your baby's coordination.

Suzy's Program

Second through third month: repeat sequence 8 times

Fourth through fifth month: repeat sequence 12 times

Sixth through eighth month: repeat sequence 16 times

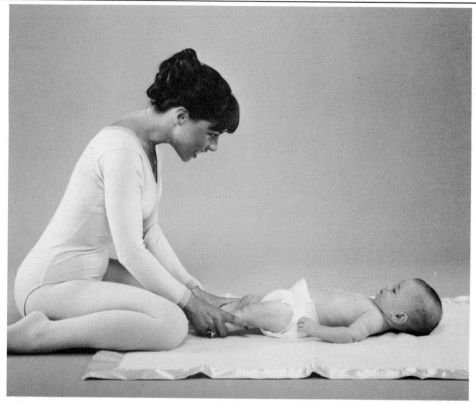

1

Place your baby on its back. Clasp your baby's legs and hold them so that they are straight.

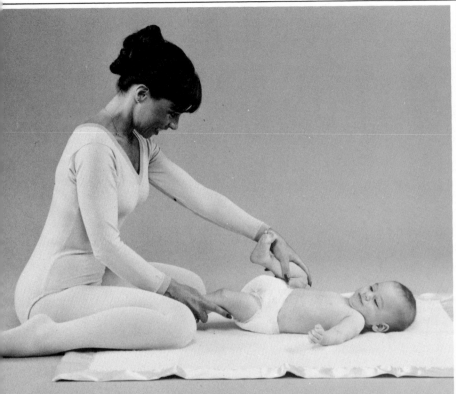

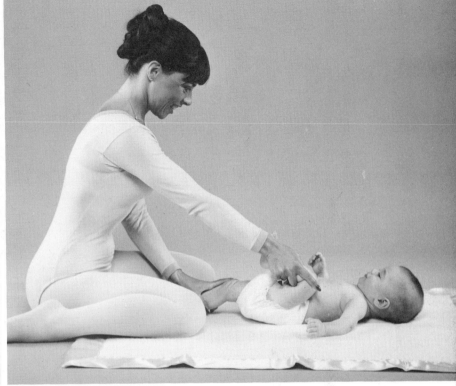

2

Bend your baby's right leg
with the knee over its
chest, keeping the left leg
straight.

3

While straightening your
baby's right leg, bend the
left knee over the chest.
Make sure that the
movements are smooth
and gentle.

Frog Swim

Although this exercise will not necessarily cause your baby to crawl at an unusually early age, it will help to make sure that your little crawler uses muscles as they should be used. After several weeks of this exercise, some babies begin to push themselves forward in little spurts.

Suzy's Program

Second through third month: repeat sequence 4 times

Fourth through fifth month: repeat sequence 6 times

Sixth through eighth month: repeat sequence 8 times

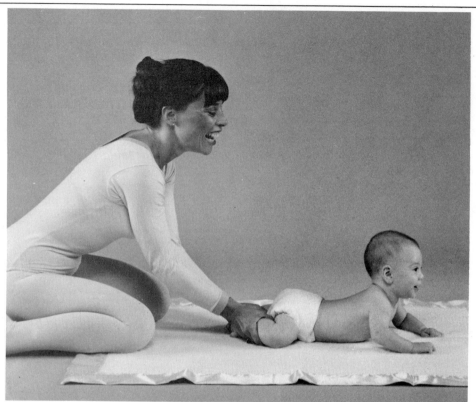

1

Place your baby on its stomach and hold its legs above the ankles. Gently push your baby's feet up toward its crotch, keeping its legs on the floor.

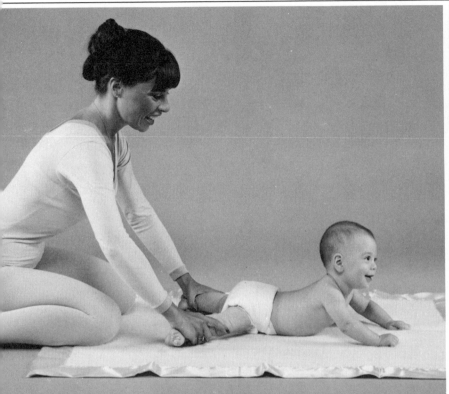

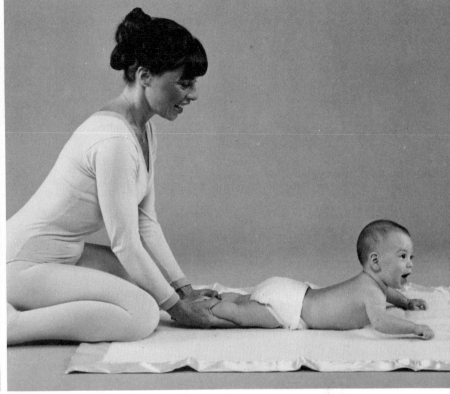

2

Straighten both of your
baby's legs so that they
are spread as far apart as
comfortable on the floor.

3

Bring your baby's legs
together, keeping knees
on the floor.

Leg and Arm Touch

This particularly active exercise has proven effective in eliminating crankiness. It is absorbing and accelerates the development of coordination.

Suzy's Program

Second through third month:
repeat sequence 4 times

Fourth through fifth month:
repeat sequence 6 times

Sixth through eighth month:
repeat sequence 8 times

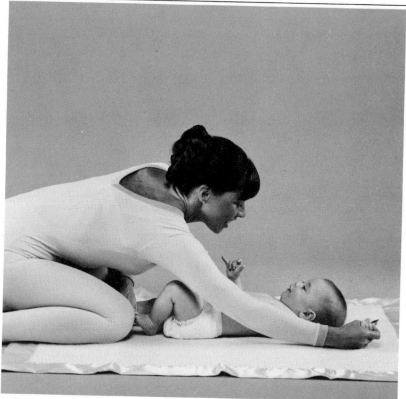

1

Place your baby on its back. Take your baby's left hand in your right hand and its right foot in your left hand.

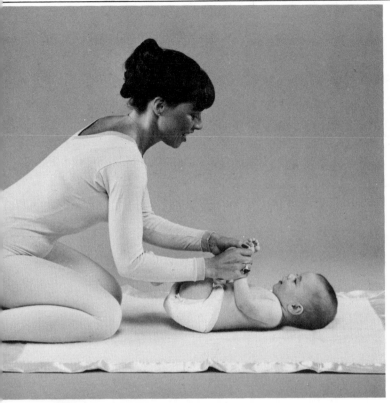

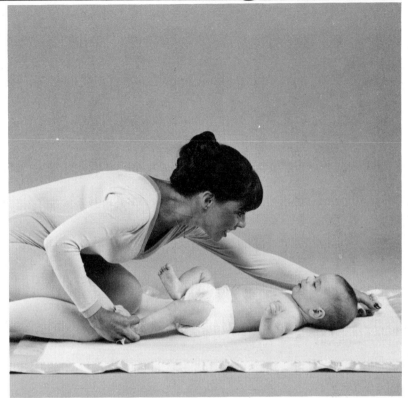

2

Bring your baby's right foot up as you bring down your baby's left hand so that they meet above your baby's torso.

3

Straighten your baby's arm and leg and repeat with the other arm and leg.

Straight Feet

This exercise has often proven effective in helping correct mild cases of pigeon toes or duck feet. If your baby has pigeon toes, turn the foot outward more often than inward. If your baby has duck feet, turn the feet inward more often than outward. During this exercise, be sure that baby's leg is held still and that only the foot moves. If you use this exercise in a remedial manner, check with your doctor.

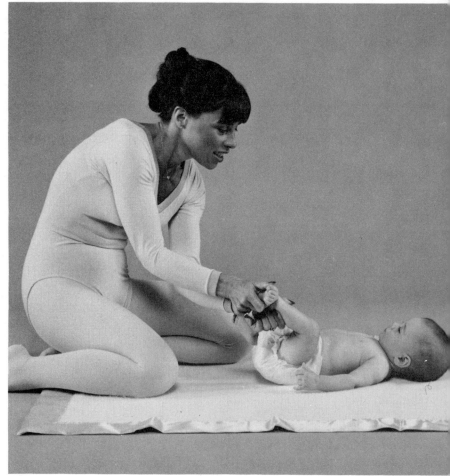

1

Hold your baby's left leg with your left hand. Place your right thumb on the ball of your baby's left foot with your fingers holding the outside of the foot. Keeping your baby's leg still, gently turn the foot outward.

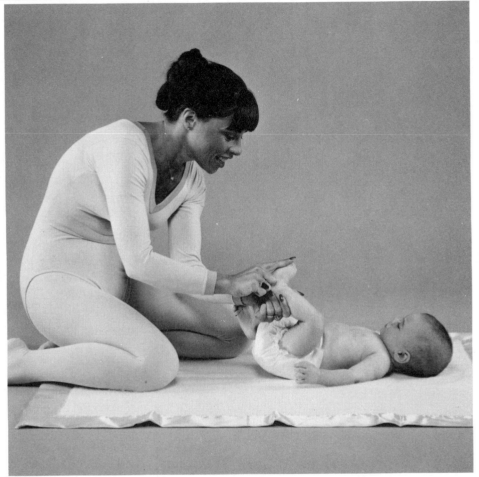

2

While pressing the outside of your baby's foot, gently turn it inward.

Suzy's Program

Second through third month: repeat 4 times with each foot (or whenever you change the diaper, if done remedially)

Fourth through fifth month: repeat 6 times with each foot (or whenever you change the diaper, if done remedially)

Sixth through eighth month: repeat 8 times with each foot (or whenever you change the diaper, if done remedially)

Wiggly Feet

In doing this exercise be sure to hold your baby's leg perfectly still. Only the foot should move.

Suzy's Program

Second through third month: repeat twice with each foot

Fourth through fifth month: repeat 4 times with each foot

Sixth through eighth month: repeat 6 times with each foot

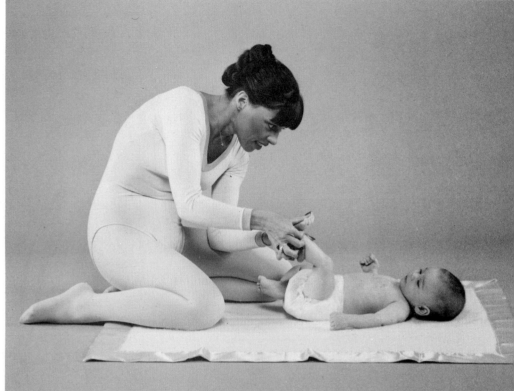

1

Place your baby on its back. Hold your baby's left leg in your left hand. Place the fingers of your right hand across the instep and your thumb on the ball of the foot. Gently push your thumb up so that your baby's foot is in a slightly flexed position.

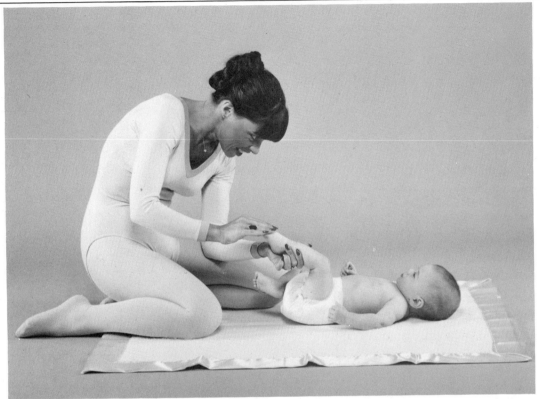

2

Release the mild pressure
exerted by your thumb
and gently press down
with your fingers so that
the foot is slightly pointed.